Praise from Readers for "Out of the Inferno"

"What happens when cancer takes center stage? Randy Evans bares his soul and shares his and Laurene's story and the aftermath of that story in this very engaging book. He combines down home Texas culture with a running commentary on lessons learned, all within the context of a trip through hell *(Dante's Inferno)*. But he continues on, out of hell, and into a new life. A powerful story."

—Linda Yarger, Medical Librarian, UNIVERSITY OF TEXAS MD ANDERSON CANCER CENTER, and breast cancer survivor

"A beautifully written memoir filled with stunning stories, terrific insights, and first-hand advice. I laughed and wept, openly and honestly dozens of times."

—Wade Rouse, bestselling memoirist and author of THE CHARM BRACELET *(St. Martin's Press)*, written under the pen name Viola Shipman as a tribute to his grandmother.

"Hearing Evans' public reading was emotional, there was not a dry eye in the room. Then everyone was laughing out loud. I was till misty-eyed reading the book. Hearing the honesty and imagining his challenge to recount that period with his family makes chapters that must be finished before putting the book down."

—Dylan Valade, President, SUNGEM

"…a deeply moving memoir that chronicles his wife's passing from breast cancer."

—Al Sevener, HUNGRY HOLLOW FILM STUDIOS, LLC

"OUT OF THE INFERNO struck close to home, almost too home, having lost my husband to cancer. He got it all: the shock of diagnosis, the hopeful efforts towards an elusive cure, and the acceptance of the inevitable finality of death. Read and feel. It will shake out your emotions and hang them up to air."

—Anne Kelly, Freelance Writer, spouse caregiver

"With epigrams from Dante, Evans details the decade long struggle of his wife's cancer. The memoir is an honest close-up of the grief Evans says triggered his return to writing. As well as the poignant and the painful, there is also the uplifting."

—Glen Young, *PETOSKEY NEWS AND REVIEW, teacher, writer*

Out of the Inferno:

A Husband's Passage Through Cancerland

Red Sky Anthology, Book 2

Randy Evans, PhD

Includes research on how breast cancer survivors manage quality of life

Copyright © 2016 Randy Evans, PhD

ISBN: 978-1-63491-435-2

All rights reserved. No part of this publication may be reproduced, stored in a retrieval system, or transmitted in any form or by any means, electronic, mechanical, recording or otherwise, without the prior written permission of the author.

Published by BookLocker.com, Inc., Bradenton, Florida.

Printed on acid-free paper.

BookLocker.com, Inc.
2016

First Edition

BLOG: randyevansauthor.com

Dante Alighieri Inferno epigraphs from a contemporary translation by Mary Jo Bang (Graywolf Press, 2012)

The first fifty pages of this book were excerpted in Red Sky Anthology: Reading Out Loud in Northern Michigan, First Edition, Red Sky Series, Book 1 (2016), Little Traverse Press.

Later chapters in this book refer to Randy Evans's research published in his doctoral dissertation, "The Zig-Zag Road: A Multi-Ethnic Study of Breast Cancer Survivor Quality of Life" (2007) ProQuest Information and Learning Company (UMI Number: 3214103)

Cover photograph by Mike Schlitt, Visions of Mike

In memory of Laurene (1947-2002) and for the brave and courageous men and women who live and work with chronic illness.

Other books by Randy Evans

Red Sky Anthology*: Reading Aloud in Northern Michigan, Red Sky Series, Book 1—published January 15, 2016, Little Traverse Press/BookLocker.com ISBN: 978-1-63491-121-4.*

Available at BookLocker.com or from your favorite online or neighborhood bookstore.

Crooked River*: Love, Adventure, and a Search for Belonging in Northern Michigan, Red Sky Series, Book 3—coming soon*

The Lawnmower Club*: How Leo Zitzelberger Lost and Found Paradise on Earth, Red Sky Series, Book 4—coming soon*

Preface

I can't remember why, but a month after my wife died from breast cancer, I visited the patient records department at MD Anderson Cancer Center in Houston, Texas. If anything, returning was an act of love or sacrament. For hours, awash in the day-imitating light of overhead fluorescents, I reviewed her medical file, a three-foot high edifice built of notes and records, placed for me in a wheelchair. The tall stack sat upright like a paper-made person. I sifted through the clinic notes and records going back over ten years to the day when Laurene had been diagnosed. The facts became palpably alive, and took the form of a story. I thought about how much I had learned, and how much love and empathy I had developed for those who suffer chronic illness.

When I took my first research course in a doctoral program three months later, I chose a topic that I would follow for the next three years: the quality of life of breast cancer survivors. I had intended going back to school in my fifties as a new chapter in my life, but living as a husband caregiver had become how I had defined myself for so long that I couldn't seem to turn the page. After I completed my dissertation, the story continued through creative writing—essays, poetry, short stories, drama, and novels about love and loss—mostly based in northern Michigan, my new home. However, burying my thoughts and feelings in the grounded disciplines of research or the fairy powers of fiction didn't bring closure. The story still followed me.

Then one day in a quiet moment, I realized that finding closure was no longer important. My daily grief still lingered, but began to soften like the lovely sunlight filtering down through the leaves and branches of the tall magnolia tree that had stood in the front yard of my Houston house.

I no longer needed to shed a burden in order to move on. I no longer wanted to get over anything. In fact, I finally understood how my loss had tied me in beautiful ways to others. My passage into and out of a Cancerland inferno had become an abiding part of me. Also, my story had become not my unique story, but the universal human story that we all share, a story that I wanted to tell to others and not forget. Funny, sad, messy, grand, and whirling with life.

1.

*Stopped mid-motion in the middle
Of what we call our life…*

Dante's Inferno, Canto I

On a rainy November day in central Texas, Neil Schmitt, my father-in-law, trudged wearily down a country road along Pecan Bayou. A tall, lean man, he bent his head against the rain. He wore a floppy hunting cap, thread-bare coveralls, and worn-out boots that he knew he couldn't afford to replace. After walking out to the road from the old tool shed that he used as a blind, he decided that he was done with hunting for good, just like that. Once Neil made up his mind to do something or not to do something, that was it. He quit smoking that way. He quit playing poker that way. And this cold, drizzly day, he decided to stop hunting.

In his seventies, I guess he had become tired of getting up before dawn to sit on a folding chair for hours waiting for a deer to show up, and also his reasons might have had something to do with unpleasant memories of the land. The days alone in the blind might have given him too much time to think about what had happened there during his boyhood—abandonment by his father, the long illness and death of his mother, and the struggles of subsistence living in a tin and tar paper shack with a dirt floor. He carried his rifle close to his body, cradled in his arms. The strap of an Army-green canvas bag hung over his wide sloping shoulders like a sack of memories.

As Neil made his way down the wet black road towards Irene Brown's house, he stopped mid-stride, and walked to the gate at Jordan Springs Cemetery where Laura, his mother, lay buried. She had died of breast cancer in the 1940s. As the sole caregiver for his mother, her long illness and death had flattened Neil's teenaged life like a bulldozer.

He rested his gun on the cyclone fence, and stepped inside the grounds. He passed by the gravestones of long-dead, half-forgotten people whom he had known during his life in Brown County, Texas. On the far side of a hundred-year-old oak tree, he removed his shapeless cap, and stood over his mother's grave. The face of the gravestone never changed. For him, it must have been like looking at a memory that couldn't be weathered away by rain or bleached out by the hot Texas sun.

Cold rain dripped on his thin gray hair, and ran down his forehead and neck. He fastened his top button, and pulled his bare hands into his coat sleeves. The air smelled of wood smoke. After about five minutes, he tapped the toe of his boot gently on his mother's flat gravestone, and returned to the road. Dogs barked from the ranches. Windmills groaned.

A Husband's Passage Through Cancerland

Jack rabbits stood by the side of the road like marbled statues. Stella, his wife, and Irene Brown, the widow of Dennis, his best friend, waited down the road at Irene's house with hot coffee, ham and eggs, biscuits and gravy. Irene had stoked the kitchen fireplace with bone-dry mesquite. Struggling down a rainy country road towards people you love, warm food, hot coffee, and a bright fire made what Neil called a life. A cure for gray thoughts on a gray day.

After I married Neil's daughter, he gave me his scoped hunting rifle. Even though the stock had been beat up with use, the gun looked well-maintained. I could tell Neil was proud of his rifle.

"I've killed a lot of deer with this pump," Neil said. "I want you to have it, because my hunting days are over." He didn't feel the need to explain.

Other than shooting a twenty-two at scout camp when I was a young boy, I had never fired a rifle. It pleased Laurene to see her father give me one of his most prized possessions. She wanted us to love each other. After a while, we did.

I took the rifle home to Grand Rapids, and didn't give it another thought until a friend invited me to go hunting in Texas the following year. Laurene and I decided to fly down to Houston where she could stay with her parents while I hunted on a lease in the Texas Hill Country. Neil and Stella were always happy to see their only daughter, and they seemed happy to see me, too. Stella had prepared chicken and dumplings for our evening meal. The steaming chicken broth smell made you want to gulp the thick air inside their tiny house. For dessert, Stella had baked a German Chocolate Cake, one of my favorites.

Neil's eyes lit up when I told him I had brought his deer rifle with me. As soon as we could be excused from the dinner table, we cleaned the gun together in the garage. The garage door was open, and a blue twilight descended on the neighborhood. On the broken-up sidewalk, people with their dogs walked slowly by and gently nodded in our direction. Neil moved his hands gently over the stock like he was touching the arm of an old friend. After we finished with the gun, he rubbed the back of his neck with a bandana, and gave me some hunting tips while he looked out the garage door to the street. He had a faraway look in his eyes. From his occasional sideways glances in my direction, I think he might have been bashful about giving me advice. Giving advice was something he rarely did. He had never had a father around to give him advice. And he never had a son. But there were a few things he wanted me to know. As the sun dropped further, he flipped on the overhead florescent light.

"First thing I want to say about hunting is empty or not, think your gun's loaded, and think everyone else's gun's loaded—safety off and ready to shoot. If someone makes a mistake and points a gun barrel at you, drop to the dirt as quick as you can. You're gonna be better off embarrassed than dead. Second thing, never look at people through the scope—that's what eyes or binoculars are for. Third, when you scope a deer, the deer's gonna look much bigger than actual size. Make sure the antlers are outside the ears. Count the tines. People frown on shooting deer under eight points.

"Another thing about scopes. Look behind your target to make sure there's nothing there. If you shoot a rancher's livestock, or worse than a cow, his favorite dog, he's gonna get real upset. You have no idea how upset. Fact is, you might see him dig two holes in the ground—one for the dead animal, and one for you. I admit that's an extreme statement, but I'd save the thought. The last thing I want to say is to keep that scope away from your eyes. You've probably never heard of 'buck fever,' but that's what happens when a big buck jumps out in front of you. You put the scope up against your eyeball and pull the trigger. You don't want to do that. The old Remington kicks like a rodeo horse. I know this, because it happened to me."

After a long pause, he added, "Now you needn't worry about getting a deer on your first hunt. Some people hunt their entire lives without getting a deer."

We walked back into the house to play Double-Nine dominoes with Laurene and Stella. Neil looked apologetic, like he felt he had said too much.

Laurene and I wanted to do something else while we were in Texas. For six months, Laurene had been concerned about a change in her left breast. Her gynecologist confirmed that she could also feel a textural difference close to the chest wall. In May 1991, Laurene met with a Grand Rapids oncologist who said he could find no evidence of disease, but he told her that she could return in a few months if she had further concerns.

Laurene asked me if I could feel anything, but I couldn't. Nothing had appeared on a mammogram, and there had been no indications on a routine test the year before. The oncologist told Laurene not to worry. He told her that a preventative measure might be to change her diet—eat more plant-based foods, and give up chocolate. There may have been more to his advice, but I only remember the chocolate dictum. I happened to like chocolate.

I knew what would follow. That was the end of chocolate. Laurene made decisions like her father. The whole family had to stop eating chocolate, and any other food that Laurene deemed to be unhealthy. She stir-fried broccoli, and other vegetarian dishes. Organic carrots and celery replaced our favorite snack foods. Bars of real butter disappeared from our refrigerator. She threw away the hoard that I had concealed behind the oatmeal in the pantry, leftover candy from Halloween.

Fruit bowls decorated the kitchen counter, inviting us to eat apples, bananas, pineapples, and grapes, rather than cookies and ice cream. Laurene purchased a blender that roared like a jet engine, as fruits and veggies were ingested, and then pulverized into green smoothies that glowed on the counter top like magical potions from a Harry Potter novel.

New cookbooks stood like scolding health foodies shouting out slogans from the kitchen book shelves—EAT KALE AND YOU CAN'T FAIL! SALADS AND BEETS ARE HEALTHY TREATS!

We stopped going out to dinner at fried food restaurants. I began to have nighttime food dreams about hot juicy burgers and crisp onion rings loaded with salt and hot fat; fish and chips slathered with malt vinegar. You know you're in trouble if you walk into a restaurant and see no catsup and mustard bottles standing around.

I took advantage of lunch in the middle of the work day to satisfy my unhealthy food cravings. I packed emergency Snickers Bars in my briefcase. When alone in the kitchen, I stuffed the jet engine with scoops of ice cream, and squeezed heavy crisscrosses of chocolate syrup on top, then added whole milk and powdered malt. Flipping the switch for a few seconds at 200 miles per hour liquefied a shake with a whisper of sound.

Our daughters concocted eating strategies of their own—for example, the Lucky Charms pitch:

"Mom, Lucky Charms are high in zinc."

"That's interesting, Meredith, how do you know?"

"It says so on the box! See, Mom."

"How much sugar?"

"14 grams."

"That's a lot of sugar, Meredith."

"But Lucky Charms also contains *mayonnaise*."

"You mean *manganese*."

Laurene loved rules to, and when she made new rules, we all had to get in line. Further, Laurene believed that if you followed the rules, life would be fair to everyone and all would be well. Her parents had raised to her to follow rules covering every aspect of daily living. Rather than ten commandments, hundreds existed.

Laurene told me that when she was a young girl, she would argue with Neil and Stella about changing the rules, but she would never break them on her own. She loved to argue, and since she was the only child, she argued most of the time with her parents, her father more than her mother. Neil once told her, "Laurene, if you argue with people like you argue with me, no one will ever like you."

Laurene made another appointment in August 1991, and again the doctor observed nothing. She returned in October, and finally the doctor noted a difference in her left breast. He said there was no cause for alarm. We wanted a second opinion, but at first, he first refused to write a letter. He looked up at us from the paperwork on his desk as if we were making a lot of trouble over nothing. When we pushed back, he reluctantly wrote a referral letter to MD Anderson in Houston. The last line of the letter read: "I don't feel this is a malignancy, but it should be biopsied to make sure."

To this day, the doctor's letter rests at the bottom of Laurene's permanent medical file at MD Anderson (PATIENT #114148). During the next ten years, I would often ferry her file from one appointment to the next to expedite appointments. After ten years, I had to move the records around the clinic in a wheelchair. The file had grown to three feet high, held together with binder clips and rubber bands; filled with blood work reports, doctor's clinic notes, radiologists' reports, imaging results from CT, MRI, and PET scans, ECG's, medications and dosages, and lab notes showing weight, temperature, and blood pressure readings. Today scanners digitize many of the details and store them neatly in computer memory, rather than the dog-eared, ragged pile of paper that multiplied like an overgrown bush into a barely-containable jumble.

We made an appointment at MD Anderson for the Monday after my weekend hunt—November 6, 1991. On the sunny fall day before the appointment, Neil, Stella, and Laurene picked me up at a gas station where my hunting buddies had dropped me off near Johnson City in Blanco County, about fifty miles west of Austin, and just south of the limestone escarpments of the Pedernales River. The Perdernales was well known for its raging flash floods, but this day, the river flowed tranquilly towards Lake Travis.

Neil stuck his head out of the car window, and said, "Howdy...did you get your buck?"

His blue eyes brightened and he laughed with his entire body when I told him that I had taken two bucks with his rifle. He kept saying, *"Two bucks! Two bucks!"* I sat in the back seat of his blue Chevy Impala with Laurene, and apologized to everyone because I stunk from not bathing for three days. Laurene wanted to know about the red crescent wound beneath my purple right eye. Contrary to Neil's warnings, when the first buck jumped out from behind a pile of brush, I had placed the scope against my eye and pulled the trigger. Just like that! Blood spewed all over my clothes and onto the ground. I thought, *did the deer in Texas shoot back?*

Neil talked freely in the car, something he rarely did. He jabbered about how he had been to Canada, and had hunted birds in South Dakota, but had never been to Michigan. With a twinkle in her eyes, Stella added that when the Canadian border guard had asked Neil for his country of origin, he replied TEXAS! Stella had been mortified. Neil questioned me about the weather in Michigan, and the hunting and fishing. He exhausted his knowledge of Michigan by telling about his general practitioner. "My doctor grew up in a town called Kalkaska, Michigan— 'three 'A's and three 'K's,'" he said slowly and repeated, "three 'A's and three 'K's—Kalkaska, Michigan. How 'bout that?"

I asked Neil why they had moved from Brownwood to Houston soon after Laurene's birth. "We wanted a better life. I didn't want to stay somewhere that was going nowhere. After the war, there were plenty of good-paying jobs in Houston. With Stella's teaching and my job with the city, we bought a house and paid for Laurene to go to college. I paid that house off in four years, because I couldn't stand the mortgage hanging over our heads. We could've been happy in Brownwood, but we did better for ourselves in Houston. Until a while ago, we kept a small apartment in Brownwood for spending weekends with our old friends. We hunted on Saturday mornings, danced on Saturday nights, and drove home after church on Sundays. Laurene came along. I expect we made the best of two worlds."

Neil entertained us with stories of Laurene's childhood, and about his friends in Brownwood. He talked about his only trip to Europe. Dennis and Irene had traveled with them, and Dennis had teased Neil for bringing canned goods to Paris. Neil justified himself by saying that he didn't know what the food would be like over there, so he had packed a few cans of red beans. On their honeymoon, Neil and Stella had invited Dennis and Irene to accompany them on a trip to "Old Mexico." Over the five-hour drive, Neil, Stella, and Laurene gave me an extensive history of their family and friends, and the stories behind each of them. I could tell how absorbed this small family was in the lives of the people they loved.

Halfway back to Houston, we stopped for a barbecue lunch at Meyer's Elgin Smokehouse in Elgin, Texas. The sign over the door read REAL TEXAS REAL GOOD. Another sign read WE HAVE THE CURE FOR NOBRISKETOSIS. In the middle of the round tables inside sat paper towel holders and large bottles of house-made barbecue sauce. The rough brick and wood walls displayed framed pictures of rodeo riders and oil rigs. Deer and antelope mounts guarded the door frames. A meat case advertised JALOPEÑO AND CHEESE SMOKED PORK AND BEEF SAUSAGE. The restaurant menu on the wall listed nearly all of Laurene's forbidden foods in one large display behind the long counter. The menu sign described a range of combinations that excited me beyond description:

BAR-B-Q BEEF, BAR-B-Q SPARE RIBS, CHOPPED BAR-B-Q BEEF, BAR-B-Q GERMAN SAUSAGE, BAR-B-Q CHICKEN, CHICKEN FRIED STEAK, FRIED SHRIMP, BQ SAUCE, HOT ROLLS, RED BEANS, POTATO SALAD, GREEN BEANS, MASHED POTATOES, COLESLAW, CORN, CARROTS, BLACKBERRY, CHERRY, PEACH COBBLER, BANANA PUDDING, SWEET TEA, AND DR PEPPER.

At hunting camp, I had started each day two hours before first light with a long walk to a brush blind. In my backpack, I had two cans of Coke and two apples to last me until an hour after sundown. Under the large PLACE ORDER HERE sign, I ordered sliced beef with pickles, onions and jalapeños on white bread with extra barbecue sauce, beans, coleslaw, and sweetened ice tea. Behind the counter, a young man who held a long flat-nosed knife sliced a long slab of smoked beef ribboned with fat. (I'm not done telling you about this meal.) For dessert, I had blackberry cobbler topped with Bluebell Ice Cream. Laurene gave me a spoonful of her banana pudding.

I remember how happy we all were. No one talked about the appointment the following morning.

When Laurene objected to my extensive food order, Neil defended me: "I've been eating like this my entire life, and I'm doing just fine. Besides, Randy killed his first deer. This is a celebration!" Shooting your first deer in Texas is a big deal like in a lot of places, but I suppose in Texas it's a bigger deal like everything else there.

After lunch, Laurene and I traded seats with Neil and Stella. I took the wheel, and drove the rest of the way back to Houston. We traversed three of Texas' geographic regions: the rolling plains of Central Texas, the Hill Country around Austin, and as we approached Houston, the Gulf Coastal Plain. From the 610 Loop we could see the skyline and the urban core of Houston, our next day's destination. I reached for Laurene's hand. I began to worry:

What tests will they do?
How long before we see the results?
What if Laurene has cancer?
How will she react?
I need to find a pen and notepad.
She looks so healthy.
She's too young to have cancer.
She follows all the rules of healthy living.
She can't have cancer.
Please, God, don't let her have cancer.

It was half dark when we pulled into the driveway. Seed carriers from the neighbor's box elders helicoptered over the concrete. Neil's camper-topped red pickup rested at an odd angle outside the garage, sporting a flat tire.

"I need to sell that truck," he said. A week later, he sold his truck. Just like that.

"Daddy's getting older," Laurene said. "I can't believe he's decided to give up hunting. I can't believe he's selling his truck."

Out of the Inferno

LESSON ONE

It doesn't matter how good you happen to be, or how well you follow the rules. Bad things can happen. There is no limit to how many bad things can happen.

2.

Not an uncommon occurrence. It makes even
The well-intended scurry like an animal
Who sees a monster in the margin of his
*   nightmare.*

Dante's Inferno, Canto II

We had been in the hospital for less than two hours on the following Monday morning. Technicians and nurses had administered an ultrasound and fine-needle aspiration of the breast. After they numbed her breast with local anesthetic, Laurene said that she only felt pressure. Twenty minutes later, a nurse told us to make another appointment for the same day. Since it had taken weeks to schedule the tests, the short interval until the next appointment frightened us.

While Laurene was getting dressed, I chased the nurse down in the hallway. She wouldn't tell me what she knew, but I could tell from the way she turned her face away from me that this was not going to be a good day.

The hours before the afternoon appointment dragged. We drove back to Neil and Stella's house, and spread a blanket out in the backyard. I can't remember what we talked about, but it wasn't about cancer. We might have talked about fire ants when one stung me, or about Neil's prolific okra garden with stalks that grew above the wood-slatted fence along the side of the house. At one point, Neil came into the backyard and trimmed some okra with his slender pocket knife. "For dinner," he said in a raspy voice. He walked back inside bent forward. I could tell he was worried. He looked like a walking question mark. When we re-entered the house, we found Stella attacking the kitchen floor with her broom, her arthritic hands wrapped around the broom handle like claws with the thumb of her left hand lower and pointed towards the floor.

Returning to MD Anderson in the afternoon, I dropped Laurene off at the entrance and drove off to park the car. I was driving Neil and Stella's car, so I looked for a wide space on the roof deck of the garage. When I approached the clinic building, I passed a dozen patients sitting outside smoking, hunched over men hooked up to IV stands like old chairs sitting next to floor lamps. A year later, the clinic would ban smoking on the premises, but I remember those emaciated men puffing away, and my thoughts at the time. *They had brought cancer on themselves. It was their fault. You'd think they'd have had enough sense to stop smoking.*

Created in 1941 as part of the The University of Texas System, MD Anderson sprawls across 25 buildings covering 14 million square feet on more than seven acres, including an inpatient pavilion with 507 beds, five research buildings, three outpatient clinic buildings, two faculty office buildings, a proton radiation clinic building, and a patient-family hotel. Within the walls, 20,000-plus cancer fighters treat 150,000 patients per year. The outpatient clinics have the feel of a busy international airport with all ages and nationalities—Arab women wearing burqas and tunics, Hasidic Jewish men with long beards and skull caps. You can pick up accents from faraway regions, like all the species of birds in the world are chirping at once, each song entering the song of another.

Christmas cards created by children cancer patients through the Children's Art Project were for sale in the lobby, as well as sparkling Christopher Radko glass-blown tree ornaments. The clinic impressed me as an upbeat place of hope, a mix of disabled and able-bodied people moving around with purpose—four to five thousand visits a day. I passed through the vast clinic lobby and found the sign for the correct elevator (ELEVATOR B).

When I arrived at the radiation clinic waiting room, Laurene sat reading a book with great intensity. She always read when she wanted to get her mind off something. Her feet were tucked under the rest of her body like she always did when she was reading. The receptionist gave us a nod within fifteen minutes. At the time, I could not appreciate that fifteen minutes was lightning fast for a cancer appointment. On clinic days, oncologists would often meet with fifteen or more patients. Some visits took a few minutes; others lasted up to an hour. It depended on what was happening with the patient. Good news. Bad news. No news.

A young radiologist in a white lab coat didn't hesitate to tell us what we had to hear. Laurene had cancer. For a moment, there was a shuddering quiet.

The doctor told us what he knew so far. The biopsy had revealed a high grade tumor (high grade refers to the aggressiveness of the tumor). The diagnosis was breast cancer (later on a pathologist who looked at the biopsy gave us a more specific diagnosis: invasive ductal carcinoma). The doctor told us that the staging, although tentative, was not the worst news we could have received, but not good news. I felt blood flushing my face and churning through my body. The tiny room seemed without air.

The TNM staging system (T=tumor, N=nodes, and M=metastasis), indicated stage 3 cancer (T3, N1, M0). At last, we knew more about what we were dealing with. T3 referred to the size of the tumor (1cm =.39 inches), and the doctor was guessing that the tumor in Laurene's left breast was more than 5 centimeters. I did the math—about two inches. N1 meant that positive lymph nodes were most likely present. M0 indicated that further testing would be required to make sure that the cancer had not metastasized to other parts of the body, since the initial diagnosis had been based on a microscopic view of the breast cells aspirated by the biopsy.

My initial reaction was shock and anger. I felt like a star was coming apart before my eyes.

Damn that doctor in Grand Rapids! What he had failed to identify over a six-month period, MD Anderson had identified in a few minutes, or at least, in a few hours.

I held Laurene's hand. Everything grew strange. I felt as though a monster had entered the room. I wanted to run away; scurry for cover. I didn't want to be there. This couldn't be happening. My eyes blurred. The objects in the room seemed out of scale. The room appeared overly small for such enormous news, a *roomette* rather than a room. We were sitting in this miniature-sized living room. The chairs and table seemed too small. The lamp looked too small for the table. The inspirational posters on the walls shouted messages that were out of place in this setting.

Unlike the smallish furniture, the posters appeared as large as billboards on a highway: CANCER IS A WORD NOT A SENTENCE, CANCER CANNOT EAT AWAY PEACE, LOVE IS BETTER THAN ANGER, MAMMOGRAPHY SAVES LIVES.

Out of the Inferno

This must be the bad news room. Are we supposed to read the posters, and think that everything is okay? They have staged this to look like someone's living room. Living room. Ha! I don't like this room, and I don't like this doctor. His lab coat with his name embroidered on the front makes him look like a garage mechanic.

Other than my grandfather, cancer had never raised its ugly head in my immediate family. Cancer happened to acquaintances or strangers, but not to someone close. Not to my parents or my children or my wife. Our marriage had just begun four years earlier. What would happen to us? Our children? I slouched down in the tiny chair.

Look at Laurene! She's doing better than me. I'm leaning back and she's leaning forward. She's leaning into the news. Her face is bright and her eyes look like clear water over stones. She wants to know the new set of rules so she can challenge them. She's making the doctor sweat under his white lab coat. She's asking so many questions! Too many to be polite. If you ask the doctor too many questions, he won't like you.

Laurene responded like she was in GE business meeting. She didn't care to charm the doctor. She wanted to know as much as she could about the pathology report. How invasive was the cancer? What other tests would be performed? What did the blood work show? How would we know if the cancer had spread beyond her chest? Where might it travel—to the other breast or somewhere else?

Her mind operated in think mode—no time for emotions. She wanted facts. The oncologist could only tell us that the cancer was locally advanced. He said, "It's bad, but not as bad as it could be." Laurene asked about staging. The doctor said that the pathologist had graded the cancer Stage IIB (the tumor was less than 5 centimeters with no evidence that the cancer had spread to auxiliary lymph nodes).

When the doctor started to leave, Laurene moved to block his exit. You could hear the ominous, fatalistic sound of metal hitting metal as she firmly shut the door. I inwardly laughed, because the doctor had no idea who he was dealing with. He had lost control of the meeting. Laurene had more questions. The doctor capitulated, and sat back down. Laurene sat back down. She smiled at the doctor with the natural charm of her father, the charm that had attracted to me when we had first dated.

The doctor took a deep breath. His face relaxed. He stopped sweating. His next patient would have to wait a bit longer. We discussed treatment options. When Laurene asked what we could do now, we were not expecting his answer. We thought that he might tell us about how we could be better informed, or learn about alternative cancer therapies. To our surprise, he told us to make sure that our marriage rested on a solid foundation. Cancer strains marriages, he said. We assured him that we could handle cancer like we had dealt with other life challenges— like raising a blended family, balancing our work schedules, and caring for our parents.

I resented his comments. *Are you a psychologist? So one doctor tells us not to eat chocolate, and this one wants us to go to marriage counseling? I thought these guys were supposed to be scientists!*

Neither one of us wanted to accept cancer as a threat to our marriage. We had worked too hard to put ourselves together, and to build a blended family. Later, we understood his intentions. Later, we knew what he meant. Living with cancer could either bring us closer together, or blow us apart. But at the time, we both refused to even think about how cancer might affect our marriage. We had enough to worry about. The doctor was trying his best to help us focus on what we could do something about, and with respect to Laurene's prognosis, to walk the line between optimism and despair.

Laurene looked for other ways to benefit from the doctor's advice. She got it—cancer involved more than medical issues. Living with cancer involved substantial quality of life challenges. As we headed back to the lobby, she began to form mental action plans. Her first thoughts focused on me and the family. She didn't want the disease to affect my work or the girls' school performance. She could quit her job and stay with her parents for treatments, if I could manage work and take care of the girls while she was away.

Laurene said that she was out of shape spiritually, and needed to do some work on her faith. She needed access to the latest new developments in breast oncology. She needed to join a support group, and maybe find a counselor. She wanted a new oncologist in Grand Rapids to backup her new doctors in Houston. We needed to revise our family budget without her income, and cut our expenses, and review our health care plans. Laurene knew that cancer was a big deal, before I did.

As we walked down the hallway towards ELEVATOR B, I could see her body change. Her blue almond-shaped eyes turned a shade darker. Her face muscles tensed with resolve. She was going to beat the cancer. "We can do this," she said. "You get the car. I'm going to buy Christmas ornaments for the girls." As I exited the building, I looked back at her. Her tall body bent over the display tables of ornaments. Her light brown hair hung over her face. She was a good-looking woman.

The lost souls still sat on the concrete wall as I walked out of the clinic to the parking garage. They resembled paper-thin zombies appearing and disappearing in smoke clouds. One man tapped a cigarette from his pack of Camels. When he wrapped his thin fingers around the cigarette and lit up, the pulsing embers looked as if they measured out the residual life still inside his frail body.

The man reminded me of my grandfather who had smoked unfiltered Camels. He had started his smoking career at age 14 as a Pennsylvania coal miner. At some time in his life, he had had his forearm tattooed with the tobacco company's iconic one-humped camel. (The smoky clouds from the cancer patients smelled like my grandfather.) Then one day soon after I was born, he stopped smoking and swearing—just like Neil had stopped smoking and playing poker.

But my grandfather quit too late. He developed lung cancer in his seventies when I was in my thirties. We sat on his screen porch eating my grandmother's pickled relish on a slice of white bread while he talked to me about how the brakes in cars had improved during his lifetime. He referred to the moon landing. He gave me advice to live by. The advice I remember—bend your knees when you lift, don't shovel snow with the shovel handle pointed at your privates, keep your shoes shined, and never join a church with a building campaign.

That my loving grandfather was dying of a strange disease was about all I knew at the time. Other than a great aunt who had died of breast cancer, there was no history of cancer in my family. I could only observe my grandfather's labored breathing as he lay in bed propped up by pillows. I was spared seeing his pain, and knew nothing of his fear and anxiety over the disease, but I first used the word "cancer" as the name for the disease that had killed my grandfather.

Would I lose Laurene like I had lost him, or could we beat this? How long would we need to deal with this unwanted intrusion into our busy lives? How could I take care of the kids and work while Laurene went through radiation and chemotherapy?

I didn't know much more about cancer at age forty-five than I had known from taking high school biology. I had no idea what caused cancer, how it spread from one site in the body to another, or how it could crowd out healthy cells, and, too often, kill people.

For weeks after Laurene's diagnosis, I listened to how people used the word "cancer" in everyday life. A newscaster on the TV said, "extreme groups are spreading like cancer." Another day, I heard "radical ideologies are metastasizing." "evil predator," "ruthless," "invasive," "intractable," and "mysterious" were the words used to portray cancer as an agent of death invested with magical powers. A life-threatening disease had inflated into a monster in my mind, one who was about to carry my wife away.

Out of the Inferno

Laurene didn't seem to feel the same way about cancer. If she harbored exaggerated fears similar to mine about the disease, she didn't share them with me. That we were beginning a long and difficult journey did not occur to me at the time. I had no clue that I was entering a stage of my life comparable to an all-consuming inferno. More than a bump in the road. A big deal.

A supreme interference. Unchartered territory.

LESSON TWO

People form crazy abstractions about cancer that we would never ascribe to the common cold or to the flu.

3.

At that, the pitch-dark plain shook.
Every aspect of that moment is burned in my
*　　brain:*
The cold sweat inside my clothes.

Dante's Inferno, Canto III

On the way back to Neil and Stella's house, we watched people speed by on their way home from work. High billboards and neon signs shouted advertising messages at us like GALLERY FURNITURE SAVES YOU MONEY, the slogan of a local businessman who held a fistful of cash over his larger-than-life head. The whole world seemed out-of-scale, from the miniature conference room at MD Anderson where we had received the bad news, to the furniture magnate on the billboard with his yard-wide fake smile.

Too small or too big. Out of the ordinary. No text for what we needed to do. Just large letters on large billboards.

We turned off the 610 Loop, and took the familiar turns to Neil and Stella's. Laurene remarked about how the neighborhood had both changed and remained the same since her girlhood. All the homes on the street were about the same size, one-story brick ranch houses built in the 50s. Neil and Stella's first home had been their last home. Laurene pointed out a Korean Methodist Church, a new community center, a strip mall with a video store, the favorite swing swaying on rusty chains in a rundown park, and a Texas-style French restaurant that Laurene said displayed exotic game mounts on the inside walls.

We pulled into the driveway of the tiny bungalow behind Neil's red pickup. I looked over at Laurene to see dried-up tear tracks on her face. She rubbed her eyes and pulled back her hair as she opened the screen door. I could tell that she was steeling herself to face her parents with the news. The wind was beginning to blow, and the screen door slammed behind her. I opened the door, and the door slammed again.

Laurene and I found Neil and Stella in the family room watching an old episode of Lawrence Welk. When Laurene informed them of her diagnosis, they both cried while an accordion player squeezed out a tune from the TV. The news upset Neil beyond anything I had ever seen from him. His emotions rose from a deep well within him. Perhaps life-long anxiety about Laurene's inherited risk surfaced. I'm sure he remembered the pain and suffering that his mother had endured. He may have thought about how hard it had been to care for his mother with no help.

Until she died, Neil had raised turkeys on the small farm. He had to chase them down in order to sell them in Brownwood. He would drive the turkeys to town in an old jalopy. At the time, there was no road access, so he had to drive over fields and through gates to get to the road. He had also worked in town at a bakery while going to school. Taking care of his mother had not been easy. For perhaps all of these reasons, his hard face softened in a sorrowful way. He fell into silence.

The big band played on the TV: *"Good night sweetheart, till we meet tomorrow, Good night sweetheart, sleep will banish sorrow..."*

After we watched the evening news with Neil and Stella, they retired to bed with hugs and kisses for both of us. They still looked stunned. Laurene and I were too hyped to sleep, so we rested and talked quietly in her bed. Her room had not changed since high school. The pink, frilly bedspread and hot pink cushions remained, the same drapes, lamps, nightstands, and a double bed with springs that creaked every time you made the slightest movement. In the small house the two bedrooms were separated by a tiny bathroom. We were literally less than ten feet from Neil and Stella. We could hear them snore.

It was useless to try to sleep. As we had done in the afternoon of this long day, we decided to take a blanket to the backyard. We placed it near the high stalks of Neil's okra garden where the tall plants hung over us like tassels. I could smell the moist evening air and a faint scent of Laurene's perfume. We reclined on our backs and watched the stars in silence. The face of the night sky dwarfed the little house in the little yard. It made me think of the lyrics, *the stars at night are big and bright, deep in the heart of Texas.* What was deep in my heart at this moment? Like the night sky, my heart contained boundless details with no specificity. All the thoughts were bumping against each other. Laurene leaned into my side, and splayed her left leg over my right leg. A soft wind blew her hair in my face. Laying on the blanket beside my wife, her face splashed by moonlight, I forgot for a moment about the cancer cells hidden under her skin.

We lay still next to each other for a longtime until I heard tapping sounds moving from place to place on the other side of the high wooden fence that enclosed the yard. What I first thought were dead leaves stirred by the wind, sounded nervous and hostile. RATS! Laurene said. I didn't bother to wait for her. I grabbed the blanket, and bounded towards the house. Laurene laughed at my quick exit.

"You run like a damn Yankee!" she said. She knew I was skittish about all the creepy, crawly creatures in Texas.

Once inside, Laurene removed two old jelly jars from a shelf in the kitchen, and handed me one. I was in a cold sweat.

"Momma and Daddy never throw anything away," she said.

On my jar, I could see the nearly washed out music bars of "My Old Kentucky Home" etched on the glass: *"eep no more, m lady...weep no more today."* Laurene poured stiff shots of Maker's Mark into the jelly jars. The whiskey warmed me. We sat down in the family room that Neil had built in the sixties so Laurene could have parties with her friends. Around the room you could see a gun cabinet, a large deer mount, a window air conditioner, and a Dad of the Year plaque that Neil had received from Laurene's sorority at Sam Houston State. After a few sips, Laurene wanted to talk.

"I am so sorry you have to deal with this. We just got married a few years ago."

"I'm glad you decided to marry me."

"I hope your girls know how much I love them."

"We all love each other."

"I'm not used to being sick. I might get ornery."

"I doubt that will happen...but you can be ornery. I won't mind."

"Don't leave me."

"I won't leave you."

We had dated for three years before our marriage; a long time from my perspective. Laurene had wanted a guarantee that our marriage would work. She didn't want to make a mistake about us. We had both been divorced after fifteen-year first marriages.

One morning, I ran across a woman from church in the supermarket who told me that Laurene had called her to do a reference check on me. I thought, *how many women do reference checks on prospective husbands?* The woman wanted me to know that she had given me a thumbs up. She examined a cantaloupe in the produce aisle—pressing the skin, smelling the stem. She lifted the melon up and down as she spoke with an accent that reminded me of Laurene's, her thoughts strung loosely together like multi-colored beads on a string bracelet.

"Don't worry, Laurene will get off the fence sooner or later. My husband says she's too intense, but I don't see her that way. She's a hard-working woman raising those two girls, holding down a job, and going back to school. I remember when John and she broke up. She jogged through the neighborhood every day crying her eyes out. She looked thin as a scarecrow. Did you know I grew up in Texas, too? I brought her a bottle of Jack Daniels after John left. She invited me in for a drink, which I expected she would. She drinks whiskey and coke...Texans do that.

"By the way, if you plan on marrying a Texan, you better learn to dance the two-step. I think it's a good sign when a woman drinks whiskey, don't you? You're a strong man. You need a strong woman. Texas produces strong women like Laurene and me. My husband asked me why Texan women are so strong, and I told him BECAUSE OF ASSHOLE TEXAS MEN! —but in all fairness, there are asshole men everywhere...not *you* of course."

She pointed the stem end of the cantaloupe in my direction like it was her prop for an asshole.

Laurene would say, "I want you to know the *real* me. I want you to know about all my faults. I want you to know every rotten part of me." She absolutely refused for me to idealize her. Maybe she knew me better than I knew myself—how I idealized women.

Of course, the flip side of this conversation was that she wanted to know every "rotten part of *me*" as well. I told her that I lived in an introverted bubble, that I spent most of my time unaware of my surroundings, that I had difficulty doing more than one thing at a time. I told her that I was impatient, and often made decisions impulsively, that my feelings were easily hurt, and that I was too ambitious about my career to live a balanced life. (I didn't tell her the really bad stuff.)

I had no idea how to close the deal with her. After three years, I had begun to think about moving on. I began to think that I could find someone else who would be less difficult to win over, maybe someone a bit more easygoing. Then one evening I said, "Laurene, I can't give you the kind of guarantee you want. There are no guarantees. You need to make a decision." I could almost hear her thinking, *I want a guarantee that our marriage will work and we'll be together forever. He won't give me a guarantee, but I know he loves me. Can I live with that? Yes. I guess we should get married before he gets tired of waiting and dumps me.*

She had the practical mind of her father.

A month later we were engaged in the dining room of a Tudor mansion that had been turned into a supper club. We met after work. That day, Laurene had given a product planning presentation on a new GE Lighting product. She wanted to talk about work for a while to clear her mind. She knew what I was about to do, but she wanted to get everything else off her chest. I proposed, and she said yes. I slipped a sapphire and diamond wedding ring on her finger. After several visits to a local jeweler, he had designed the ring to Laurene's specifications. She had wanted a sapphire ring that looked like Princess Diana's. She knew what she wanted, and did not like surprises. That night she brought her Polaroid camera along. Pictures preceded kisses.

During our engagement, Laurene signed us up for pre-marital counseling. We enrolled in a workshop titled "Stepping into Step Parenting." A psychologist administered batteries of inventories. We discovered that our two personality types couldn't have been more different; we were what Carl Jung had named "Dionysian opposites." Laurene was an extrovert. I was an introvert. Laurene made decisions based on facts. I made gut-based decisions. Laurene used her mind to solve problems. I solved problems based on feelings and values. Laurene liked to plan the future in detail. I preferred to let things happen.

Wedding planning proved to be the first test of our significant style differences. We met every night after work to go over the invitation list, the wedding attendants, the photographer, the food and entertainment. She wanted a preacher friend to perform the service, but she wanted to write out what he would say and limit his time. We listened to tapes from local musicians, and settled on a harpist. She wanted the girls to wear identical outfits with matching white and pink hats, dresses, stockings, and shoes. We ordered both a white cake and a dark groom's cake, a Southern tradition. I chose German chocolate. What if our outdoor wedding was rained out? We needed a backup plan. The details seemed to be endless, and I would often cut off our weeknight meetings by eleven.

Out of the Inferno

During the months before the wedding, I also had to pass muster with Laurene's entire family: Jennifer and Meredith, my future stepchildren; her parents, Neil and Stella; Laurene's aunts and uncles and cousins from Texas, including her Uncle William Nesbit Rice who had spent his life bull riding on the rodeo circuit.

When I first met Uncle Rice (nicknamed W.N.) and Laurene's cousins, Bo and Billy Don, we sat in the family room with Neil while Laurene, Stella, and the other women removed dove filets from milk cartons, dipped them in milk, egg, and flour, and began to batter fry them on the stove in a cast iron skillet. No one said a word for a long time. I noticed that I was the only one sitting there without a big belt buckle and Western boots. There was no TV playing, or anything else to distract us from sizing each other up. Everyone held a tumbler of iced tea. Nothing to nibble on other than some unshelled pecans. Finally, after what seemed years, Billy Don half-turned to me, careful not to make eye contact.

"Shoot birds?"

"No, I've never shot a bird."

(Long Pause)
"We do."

I don't know how it happened, but they all decided they liked me. At least they didn't take as long as Laurene had. Billy Don and his family ended up supporting Laurene and me in many different ways over the next ten years.

We married on September 5, 1987. Amy and Laura, my two daughters, along with Jennifer and Meredith, wore frilly pink bridesmaid dresses that Laurene had chosen, along with white hats, white stockings, and white shoes. They each carried a bouquet of pink flowers while the harpist played the Pachelbel Canon in D. The preacher read his scripted sermon with only a few additional anecdotes. At the time, Amy and Laura were 13 and 11; Jennifer and Meredith, were 10 and 6. Meredith had to be pried from her mother's arms, as we left the reception. She sobbed uncontrollably. She had never been away from Laurene before.

Laurene had left the details of the honeymoon to me. I was thrilled that she would delegate our honeymoon trip to me. How uncharacteristic of her. "Surprise me!" she said. Boy, would she regret it.

When we arrived in Zurich the day after the wedding, Laurene asked me for the itinerary. I told her that I had made reservations for the first night, and rented a Fiat for two weeks. There was no itinerary. She looked surprised, but not pleased.

Out of the Inferno

I thought that we might cross the Alps like Hannibal, and roam around Italy for a few weeks. Unfortunately, I had rented a car in Switzerland that required unleaded fuel. When we crossed the border into Italy, we were provided with a map showing six AGIP stations with unleaded fuel in the entire country. When we arrived at the first station with its yellow, black, and red dragon logo, Laurene jumped out of the car with her dictionary, and towered over a short Italian gas attendant. He looked up at her with horror as if this tall American woman was about to attack him.

"S*enza piombo?*" Laurene shouted with her head pointed at the phrase section of the tiny dictionary.

"*No, no, senza piombo.*" The man raised his arms skyward, as though he was searching for divine protection.

They station was out of unleaded gas. We found gas later in the day, and stopped at a bank for *lire*. Gas, cash, and a place to sleep were Laurene's priorities until she settled down, and we started to have fun. Over the next two weeks, we stayed in all manner of lodging, from an estate home in Lucca with satin wallpaper, chandeliers and marble-walled showers, to a room in Padua with unpainted walls, peeling plaster, a bare light bulb hanging from the ceiling, and a shared bathroom down the hall.

Our honeymoon ended in an odd way. We received a call from Laurene's boss at GE. He wanted her to attend a product marketing meeting in Paris on the day she had been scheduled to return to work. He said that the company would pay for her air fare, rescheduling penalties, and expenses, if she could rearrange her return trip. So on the final day of a romantic two-week romp through Europe, Laurene flew from Milan to Paris, and I flew from Milan to Cleveland. No one was more surprised than our girls when I arrived home without their mother.

A week later, Laurene returned home, probably the only GE employee to ever be reimbursed for a honeymoon trip. Neil and Stella had been our babysitters, and they stayed on to help me out until Laurene returned.

"That was an awful lot to ask," Neil said, referring to Laurene's boss. "How in the heck did they find you?"

Laurene planned our future trips. Over the following years, we would load the kids in the car or book flights for what Laurene called their educational vacations. Laurene wanted the girls to see the country: Boston, Chicago, Hawaii, Houston, New York City, Baltimore, Philadelphia, Washington, DC, and Williamsburg, Virginia, among others, whether they wanted to or not.

Laurene would read about what we were to see while I drove the car. The girls wanted to buy trinkets in souvenir shops, and a constant stream of complaints issued from the back seat, the most common one: "Jennifer's knees are sticking to my knees!"

Once, Meredith passed her mother a note predicting that she would soon have a fit. Laurene responded by writing her a brief inquiry about when and where she intended to have her fit. Meredith replied that she would wait until we had arrived home, because the backseat was too crowded for a proper fit. Later, Meredith changed her mind, and informed Laurene that she was going to jump out of the car window, but she never did. Instead, she turned herself upside down, and through the rear view mirror, I could see her pacing off the ceiling of the car in her pink Roger Rabbit high tops.

No matter what the complaints, Laurene dragged us from one museum and historical marker to another from North to South and from one Coast to the other. Determined that the girls would grow up well-educated and well-traveled, Laurene never gave up wanting to see the world along with her family. Staying around home was her father's idea of a good life, and my father would agree. They had traveled far and wide during WWII. But for Laurene, new places were like wrapped gifts to be opened with curiosity and delight, gifts she could share with the people she loved.

The guarantee that our life together would work was something I couldn't give Laurene before our marriage, but when she asked me not to leave her after her cancer diagnosis, I gave her a promise that I could keep and wanted to keep.

LESSON THREE

When you see a clear sky, a smooth ribbon of highway ahead, and think you will keep going on and on past the horizon, all of a sudden there is no sky, no road, and no horizon. You are lost without a map.

4.

*...hearing this saddened me; I could clearly see
There were many here of great worth,
Suspended in Limbo between better and worse.*

Dante's Inferno, Canto IV

Early evening the next day, we met a kind, intelligent woman whom Laurene had contacted for information about support group meetings. She unlocked the door to THE ROSE, a mammography facility on Stella Link Road, so we could prepare for the next day's appointment with Laurene's primary oncologist. She also lent us a tape recorder to record our conversation with the doctor. Laurene thanked her for lending a tape recorder to a perfect stranger. She promised to return it.

The facility also served as the site for "Rosebuds," a support group that Laurene would later join. Rosebuds had a tall file filled with tons of information not yet available on the Internet.

Laurene looked through the file cabinet, drawer by drawer. She didn't want to miss anything. The dedicated support group room contained wigs, prostheses, and pictures of the support group members. We stayed until after midnight, looking at clinical trial information, survival statistics, and treatment options. We became thoroughly tired and confused. This was the first of many evenings and nights that I would spend in buildings at or near the Texas Medical Center, often trying to catch some sleep despite the pounding jackhammers, persistently opening space for new buildings to fight cancer.

The following day, Laurene met with her oncologist. After expressing frustration about not knowing what to do, she said, "I need you to be my advocate." He gave her a hug and said he would. Over the following decade, he consistently treated her as a woman first—a woman who happened to have breast cancer. He would begin each appointment by asking Laurene for her questions, but I could tell that his examination had begun as soon as we walked through his door. He observed how Laurene expressed herself, her tone of voice, the movement of her body. I took careful notes. Sometimes I had questions, too, and the doctor also listened to me, and answered my questions. I always felt that we were part of a team. Getting directly involved in her survival remained a constant for the next ten plus years.

Getting directly involved in her survival remained a constant for the next ten plus years. Laurene wanted information, even when the news wasn't positive. She asked so many questions, that we began to call them "Laurene questions." Her brand of questioning was sincere, succinct, appropriate, and always polite. If the answers didn't satisfy her, she asked follow-up questions. Her tone of voice was calm and unthreatening, not a hint of underlying emotion or a bit of sarcasm. In spite of her father's concern that people wouldn't like Laurene if she argued to much or asked too many questions, people liked and even loved her. But her questions were unrelenting:

How many treatments will I have?
How long will each treatment take?
Will the drugs be administered by IV?
Should I eat before treatment? After treatment?
Can I take my regular medications?
What side effects are there?
How can the side effects be treated?
Will the side effects get better or worse during treatment?
Can I still walk and ride my bike?
Will I lose my hair right away?
Would you give me your daytime phone number? Your nighttime number?
Do you have a beeper?

As a product manager at GE, attention to detail had been Laurene's strength. She absorbed facts from all facets of life, including popular culture. She knew more about sports than most men, and could trade opinions with the most avid sports fanatic. She didn't read the sports pages for fun. She regarded knowing about sports as a career strategy in a male-dominated company. Her ability to absorb facts extended beyond sports. She liked history, especially Texas history. She could name all 254 counties in Texas. One year, Laurene brought us to San Antonio where she toured us through the Alamo like a history professor taking her students on a field trip.

Laurene also knew how to get things done outside the system. From the cafeteria to the pharmacy to physical therapy to appointment scheduling to the billing department, people wanted to assist her, or assist me on her behalf. She charmed people. The staff helped everyone, but they helped her a bit more. She knew that people could help her. "The nurses are the key," she said. "Doctors are important, but nurses will answer questions the doctors can't or won't." She absorbed hundreds of names at the clinic, and more than names, she knew who people were dating, what they were studying in school, and where they grew up. When we were at home, I often overheard Laurene counseling with staff from the hospital on the telephone about everything from how to break up with a boyfriend to how to buy a car or a house.

And when she couldn't charm people, she begged. "You have to know how to beg," she told me. "No one should be above begging."

The breast oncology team recommended a delay in surgery to see if the tumor could first be reduced in size through chemotherapy and radiation.

Unconventional at the time, Laurene's case had to be presented to an Institutional Review Board. Laurene sat behind a curtain in the back of a conference room, while a panel of doctors discussed her case. She wore a hospital gown in the event one of the doctors wanted to examine her. She could hear all the deliberations. Like a jury, they reached a verdict. The doctors approved the proposed protocol, one that would later become a standard treatment option. Lopping off a woman's breasts had most often been the first procedure, rather than second or third.

Laurene's treatment began in December 1991 with neoadjuvant chemotherapy (FAC), a concoction of three powerful drugs: 5-fluoroucil (5FU), doxorubicin (Adriamycin), and cyclophosphamide (Cytoxan, C). Side effects include vomiting, diarrhea, mouth sores, loss of hair, heart problems, low granulocytes, anemia, and low platelets. After six cycles over eighteen weeks, her hair, eyebrows and eyelashes fell out, but her immune system remained strong enough to complete the regimens. Her blood counts fell after each infusion, but recovered in time for the next assault. She kept her schedule.

We attended a Bears game at Soldiers Field in Chicago later that month, and the wind from Lake Michigan blew Laurene's wig off to the astonishment of the crowd around us. We attended the game with a Chicago lawyer and his wife. He was a business associate of mine. We had chosen not to broadcast

Out of the Inferno

Laurene's diagnosis outside of our family and close friends. Needless to say, Laurene's bald head surprised the couple. Fans below us passed the wig back up the aisles like a tray of nachos. Laurene laughed, and stuffed the wig into her coat pocket. After the game, we all went to lunch, and we brought them up to date.

Laurene was a modest person, and the wig incident had humiliated her. She didn't like exposing herself to anyone, and she dreaded any form of public humiliation. She had been raised around shy people, and people who were sensitive about their education, the kind of work they did, and how they looked. She told me how Neil never went beyond the eighth grade in school, but that he had practical intelligence. She said that even though Stella had graduated from college, she didn't have much self-confidence. You didn't put people down, or push them too far. You learned to overlook minor irritations and idiosyncrasies. In her business life, she would ignore chauvinistic comments, swearing, dirty jokes, and grouching. Everyone was entitled to a bad day, and besides, confronting people was not the way to get what you wanted.

When we were first married, Laurene told me never to criticize her in public. "You can say whatever you want to me in private, but if you feel the need to criticize me in public, hold your tongue." The first time I made a public remark that Laurene deemed inappropriate, she tried to gently kick me under the table. I jumped a mile. She never tried that again. I have always been highly reactive to unexpected body contact; one reason I have never turned my cell phone on vibrate mode.

The accumulated effects of chemotherapy drugs left Laurene with nausea, constipation, and mouth sores. Her balance deteriorated to the point that when we walked together, I placed a hand under her elbow to keep her steady on her feet. Her skin felt tender and sensitive. She had difficulty sleeping. In the morning, I knew when she woke up, because she flapped her numb hands to restore circulation like a bird flapping its wings. She experienced the mental confusion and difficulty concentrating, which people call chemo brain. Normally keeping everything in her head, she started to write things down on a calendar. Her periods gradually stopped with the early onset of menopause. "At least I'll never have hot flashes," Laurene said (she actually did).

The doctor kept telling Laurene how well she was doing compared to other patients. He encouraged her to take her pain medicine. He told her that addiction to drugs was rare in cancer pain management. She tried to keep a positive attitude. She ate healthy foods, and drank plenty of water. She tried to regard the harsh chemicals flooding through her body as agents of healing rather than poison. She kept up a mantra, *"breathe, think positive, you can do it."*

Out of the Inferno

We flew back and forth from Grand Rapids for the infusions in Houston that were administered through a catheter inserted in Laurene's right forearm. We arrived early at the infusion therapy waiting room. The waiting room was smaller than most of the clinic waiting rooms, and sometimes there were no empty chairs, so patients sat in spare wheelchairs or on the floor. The wait time might range from one to six hours. Once a room opened, we might wait another hour for the drugs to arrive or for a special team to access the catheter. When the bags of drugs arrived, a nurse would read the names of the drugs and dosages to another nurse to make sure they were correct. The nurses also instructed us to keep a journal, but not the kind of journal we expected. They asked us to log in Laurene's reactions to the infusions—vomiting, nausea, diarrhea, hives, skin redness near the injection site—noting the date, time, intensity and estimated volume of each occurrence.

Long hours would pass beneath the IV tree followed by more wait time after the infusions ended. The bright florescent lights glowered above us like a stationery sun on an endless day. There was no shade under the IV tree. The drip lines could not quench our thirst. No sound to soothe us other than the soft whirr of the infusion pump. I sat beside Laurene reading, or ran errands to check on future appointments, pick up prescriptions, bring back food from the cafeteria, or work through billing problems in the finance office (I received a two-inch stack of billing statements each month). The huge complex became so familiar to me, that even I couldn't lose my way.

Some days, I walked over ten miles through the corridors. I became adept at giving people directions to remote areas in the clinic. After a while, I developed a sense that I belonged there, feeling good about having a place to be useful. I knew which way to turn after each stop on ELEVATOR B, and all the other elevators.

One day, we arrived for an eleven o'clock morning appointment that ended at two the next morning. There had been a medical emergency with one of the patients, so the entire schedule backed up. Then, Laurene's medical file disappeared. I had to retrace her prior appointments over the last week, and finally found the large file in physical therapy. Over the next ten years, Laurene would go through this chemotherapy routine at least twenty-five times—low doses once a week, high doses every three weeks. After her veins deteriorated from the arm catheter, the doctors implanted a CVC (central venous catheter) in a large vein in her chest.

In April 1992, Laurene's blood counts had recovered sufficiently from the chemo to begin five weeks of pre-op radiation therapy to her chest. She stayed with her parents in Houston, and I went back to work in Grand Rapids, and took care of the children. I learned how to be a functional cook, but since I didn't get home from work until around seven, we went out to eat at places that Laurene would not have approved, like a sports bar where the girls and I played video trivia with biker dudes while gnawing on chicken wings and ribs, our fingers and hands bright orange from the hot sauce.

The girls seemed to be doing fine keeping up with their homework, and doing fun things with their friends. Meredith had been through Montessori school, and had learned to work independently. When I asked her if she needed help, she described her schedule of assignments, but only asked for help with one project. Odyssey of the Mind Project, an international creative problem solving program, drove me crazy. The project took weeks to complete, and when the contraption we invented neared completion, Meredith performed a test run. She donned her pink gymnastics tights and found a funny pink hat to wear on her head.

With a flourish of her baton, she set off a mousetrap screwed to a wooden plank. The energy from the sprung mousetrap spun two 33 speed vinyl records that I had found in the basement. The records were attached by an axle to a carved wooden car with a needle protruding from the front of the hood. Once in motion, the wheels moved towards the end of the plank where a large inflated pink balloon cowered. The needle popped the balloon while Meredith raised her head and arms to the sky in triumph like a magician who had pulled a rabbit out of her top hat. Relieved and surprised, I clapped, cheered, and hugged her. It wasn't rocket science, but it was science.

Our daughters knew that we loved them, and that they would not be abandoned no matter what happened to their mother. One evening, Meredith and I decided to take a selfie of the two of us wearing wire coat hangers under our chins and over the top of our heads with the hooks on top like antennae. We looked like a couple of silly space aliens. We had fun. During Laurene's absences, I took care of the girls, and the girls took care of me. Laurene had been the primary enforcer of the family rules. When she was in Houston, I had to be the bad guy once in a while. For example, one day a boy roared into our driveway on his new motorcycle. He wanted to take Jennifer for a ride. Helmet or no helmet, not on my watch, she had to stay put.

Laurene developed a happy routine of riding a bicycle each morning in her parents' neighborhood. Then she would drive down to the clinic for her radiation treatments. We talked everyday on the phone about details of her appointments, including profiles of her lab technicians and other people she met at the clinic. We talked about the challenges of her aging parents. I gave her daily reports on the children and their schedules. I talked about work. Haworth allowed me to travel less, so I could be home with the girls, but managing on my own wasn't easy.

In addition to our activity reports, we discussed our ups and downs, our funny and scary dreams, and once in a while, our mutual fears that centered on side effects of the cancer—physical and mental side effects of the treatments, the emotional side effects on our relationship, the side effects on the kids and our parents. We worried that the cancer would overcome us in unforeseen ways causing our entire lives to become side effects of cancer. We constantly reassured each other that everything would be okay. Privately, we both worried about each other.

"Do you think you would benefit from some counseling?" Laurene asked.

"I don't think so, but maybe you should find a good therapist," I replied.

"I've never been to a shrink before. I'll have to do some research. I don't want a quack. Have you noticed all the signs for astrologers and palm readers we pass on Shepherd on the way to the clinic?"

"I wouldn't rule out anything. You never know, " I said. "Someday magicians might find a trick to cure cancer."

I waited in the car outside the counseling center. Laurene jumped in to report on her first therapy session. "HE TRIED GUIDED IMAGERY ON ME!"

Her tone of voice gave me the impression that the therapist had assaulted her in some way, or pushed a big red button after attaching electrodes to her skull.

"He asked me to imagine my favorite color. When I told him that blue was my favorite color, he said that the color blue was too easy. He said to imagine purple. What kind of question is that? How will a crazy question like that help me? I'm a literal person. I can't do this."

"What did you expect?" I said.

"I thought psychologists listened, took notes...then told you what to do."

"Well, did he listen and take notes?"

"Yes, but he asked me to do things I can't do...ridiculous things. How would *you* describe purple?" Laurene looked at me with lawyerly eyes, like she was cross-examining a crime witness.

"Your eyes when you're angry, the sky at sundown, frosting on a birthday cake, the skin of an eggplant, the color of hope..."

"Our brains are different."

"You need to see colors with your heart and mind."

"Easier for you than me."

When I asked her how the rest of the session went, she said that she had relaxed enough to fall asleep on the therapist's couch.

Laurene continued with the therapy for the next ten years. She not only learned to imagine the color purple, but after many sessions, she developed the ability to hypnotize herself. Self-hypnosis helped her manage extreme pain when morphine failed. Sometimes she took naps during her sessions, something she rarely did at home. Ever practical, if a therapy session was not working for her, at least the therapist had a good couch. When nothing helped, or she had a setback in her treatment, she used her most profane word, RATS!

If she was really unhappy, she would add an addition rat or two, but I don't recall her ever using any other word. I never heard Neil swear, and certainly not Stella. Against the rules.

Talking with Laurene after her therapy sessions gave me insights into what Laurene most wanted from me as her husband. Laurene wanted my presence more than anything. She did not want me to be her therapist. She rarely shared her deepest emotions with me, partly because she didn't fully understand them herself. Her definition of emotional support was helping her to get showered and dressed, driving her to and from her appointments, taking notes during our clinic sessions, communicating with the outer circles of our friends and family so she could talk with the inner circle of her friends and family. So I had the impression that she preferred to do the housekeeping of her inner life, and she wanted me to do the yard work of her outer life. I had a difficult time understanding this for a long time, but it's what she wanted, not what I thought she wanted, that counted most.

Laurene divided her world into neat categories. Doctors followed scientific disciplines and objectivity, and psychologists indulged in subjective and untested theories of human behavior and mental processes. She walked through life with right and wrong, or good and bad categories most of the time like good and evil angels rested on her opposite shoulders. While she was highly intelligent, and could understand complexities and tones of gray in situations, she did not prefer middle categories or positions. Neil was like that.

For example, Laurene divided people and animals, including the girls and me, into either critters or varmints. When I asked her to explain the difference, she told me that critters were basically harmless creatures like squirrels and rabbits. They might get into mischief in your attic, but they were inherently cute and lovable like her daughters and me when we misbehaved. On the other hand, varmints were harmful like a coyote or a fox who would dig holes in the ground to break the legs of cattle, or steal chickens from the coop. Or like the poisonous snakes that lived in the muddy water tanks in Brownwood. When she didn't like our behavior, she called us varmints.

Laurene never referred to cancer as a journey. She never referred to cancer as a battle. The truth of the story of Laurene was tied to her odyssey to return to her life before cancer, to return home from Cancerland—the constant pressure to follow regimens, reverse setbacks, discount bad news, fight the pain, look for breaks—adapting, improvising, pretending, forgiving, and never wavering from her ambition to simply live.

For her, cancer was the Great Interrupter. It was not a mysterious force, a dramatic antagonist, or the voice of God. It certainly was not a blessing in disguise to test her faith or to make her a better person. Neither was cancer a payback for wrongdoing. She didn't want redemption. She wanted a cure. Her adventure was not coming home to God, but coming back to her house in Grand Rapids and her life before cancer. That's how it was.

A Husband's Passage Through Cancerland

Lennie was delighted. "That's it—that's it. Now tell how it is with us."

George went on. "With us it ain't like that. We got a future. We got somebody to talk to that gives a damn about us. We don't have to sit in no bar room blowin' in our jack jus' because we got no place else to go. If them other guys gets in jail they can rot for all anybody gives a damn. But not us."

Lennie broke in. "But not us! An' why? Because...because I got you to look after me, and you got me to look after you, and that's why."

Of Mice and Men by John Steinbeck

LESSON FOUR

Suffering doesn't necessarily lead to redemption.

5.

I made my way down from the first circle
To the second, which has a smaller circumference
But much more misery, which makes more tears.

Dante's Inferno, Canto V

Through all this turmoil, the girls decided that they wanted a pet. Most of their friends had pets. Laurene and I talked about this subject at great length. She never turned down small or large requests from the children without careful thought. Her personal and family strategy had been to keep our lives as close to normal as possible, and to give our children the same opportunities as other children (it was only fair). How did owning a pet fit in to this strategy? *Why couldn't we simply say no?* I thought.

We decided to ease into the idea. Laurene informed the girls that they needed to start small, and prove that they were capable of caring for a helpless animal. We bought a goldfish. They forgot to feed the fish and clean the bowl. Three weeks later, Laurene found the poor little fellow floating belly up. It had died a slow and agonizing death, sucking for air on an empty stomach.

"See, you didn't care for the fish, and the poor fish died," Laurene said.

Meredith would soon regret her reply, "Mom, if the fish had been a dog, the fish would've barked for food."

Blaming the poor fish for not having vocal cords was enough to hold off another pet for a few months, but we decided that the kids needed a pet, so we bought a happy, industrious hamster who entertained us by running on his little wheel. Laurene admonished the girls about cleaning the cage, but the girls didn't clean the cage. The hamster cage smelled so foul that the girls relocated the hamster and its cage to the back porch in the dead of winter. I found the poor little creature on a Saturday morning frozen solid as a stone. At last, I thought, we were done with pets. No one wanted to take care of a pet. We were all too busy—work, school, soccer practice, ballet, gymnastics, and boys.

Then one Friday night I came home from work, and Meredith ran to me laughing and crying for joy. She hugged my leg, and thanked me for buying her a cat. Jennifer, her older sister, said, "*You dummy,* that's not our cat. I'm cat sitting for the weekend." Meredith sobbed inconsolably, as if the cat had resided in our house for years and someone was going to take it away. After starving a gold fish and freezing a hamster, the girls did not deserve a pet, but the next week, Brother Butterscotch, an orange tabby kitten, joined the family. When we told Neil about the new member of our family, he was less than enthused. "It takes a cat a long time to die," he said.

The girls took good care of Bro, and he grew into a fine big cat with a movie star personality. How big? A woman once ran away from Bro screaming. She thought she had sighted a cougar. When he entered a room, you could turn the thermostat down because of his body heat. Laurene was happy to have another cat. Her only other cat had been run over by a car in front of her house when she was a little girl.

While Laurene stayed in Houston with her parents for radiation treatments, I did the laundry as best I could. I hadn't done laundry since college. I found that my methods were not up to the satisfaction of the girls. One wash load for whites and one for darks, and one dryer setting for everything, didn't meet their standards. Meredith kept inheriting shrunken blouses from her older sisters. I thought that pink and white were close colors, but soon the white clothes looked pinkish.

I couldn't understand the settings on the washer and dryer. Why didn't these appliances simply have a pull choke, a start button, and stop switch like my lawn mower? And have you ever tried to fold girls' clothes? Nothing is rectangular. I could barely handle towels, but folding panties, bras, blouses, shorts, and tiny socks drove me crazy. It was like trying to fold a half-twisted Möbius strip. I also didn't understand why on earth you needed to fold something that you wore under something else. Who would know? Each week I noticed that my loads of laundry were smaller than the week before. I had no idea what had happened until years later. The girls had stuffed their laundry in old suitcases in the attic, hoping that Laurene would return before they ran out of fresh clothes.

One day, I had finished heaping a modest pile of dirty clothes into the washer, slammed the dryer door shut, and walked towards the kitchen to prepare supper. I was about to make one of the girls' favorite meals—slow-roasted chicken on the grill and a Caesar salad with lots of parmesan cheese and croutons. As I began to coddle an egg for the dressing, loud thumping noises sounded from the laundry room. I thought the washer had spun off balance.

No, when I wasn't looking, Brother Butterscotch had jumped into the dryer. I opened the door, and he shot out of the dryer like a fluffy canon ball. I didn't see him again for days. He had run away from home. Our next door neighbor called to inform me that Bro had appeared in her kitchen looking for food. I picked him up, and brought him home. He never entered the laundry room again. I hadn't killed the goldfish or the hamster, but I nearly killed the cat.

A Husband's Passage Through Cancerland

***

In May 1992, after completing her chemotherapy and pre-op radiation to the chest, we returned to Houston for a radical mastectomy of Laurene's left breast. The chemotherapy and radiation had not shrunk the tumor. Not one bit.

We met with the anesthesiologist and the surgeon, and after asking dozens of questions and receiving satisfactory answers, Laurene said she was ready. The operation was scheduled for the next morning. The afternoon before, Laurene picked out favorite tunes to play on her Sony Walkman before the operation. She liked music. Neil and Stella fixed chicken and dumplings for dinner while I watched. Neil cooked a whole chicken, and then Stella carefully held her arthritic hands over the steaming pot of shredded chicken and broth as she dropped in the dough for dumplings. There was nothing complicated about the recipe, but Laurene told me that she had never been able to duplicate her mother's skill with the dish, or for that matter, Stella's version of chicken-fried venison.

After dinner, Laurene wanted to go to bed early. She removed her clothes in the bedroom, but her pajamas stayed on the bed. I was puzzled, because Laurene never liked to have sex in the close quarters of her parents' small house. Was she going to make an exception this evening?

"I want you to take a picture of my breast," she said.

"I don't want to take a picture of your breast. *Why in the world...*"

"What if we change our minds about reconstructive surgery?"

"So?"

"Well, don't you think they would want to see what my old boob looked like?"

"Could be...but we don't have a camera, and even if we did, I don't think you can get pictures like that developed."

"I already thought about that."

Laurene reached into her suitcase, and pulled out the old Polaroid camera. I hadn't seen it in since the night I had asked Laurene to marry me. I thought we had thrown it away, but I should have known better. Laurene never threw anything away.

"Now don't take a picture of me. Take a picture of the breast. That's all we need. It should work. I replaced the batteries, and took some test pictures of Bro. He's such a handsome cat."

A Husband's Passage Through Cancerland

I did what I was told.

After the operation, I stood outside the door of her room in the hospital wing as Laurene returned from the operation. She rode sitting up on the gurney with an IV stand wheeling behind her. She had a big smile on her face. As she came closer, she smiled and waved to me like she was sitting on top of a parade float. Even with the IV lines and drainage tubes and the discomforts of major surgery, she knew that she had survived. She was looking forward to going home. "I've never been so happy to see you," she said. She joked about how she had never taken drugs, but when you needed them, they weren't all that bad.

The next day, her doctor entered the hospital room to inform us that eleven of seventeen lymph nodes removed from under her left arm had tested positive for cancer. That information changed her diagnosis from Stage IIB to Stage IIIB (cancer spread to nine or more auxiliary lymph nodes). The news stunned us. We had been worried that a few cancer cells might have escaped the surgeon's knife from around the borders of the breast, but we had regarded the lymph node dissection as a cautionary measure. The doctor told us that this was not a death sentence, but the news was not good. He recommended that Laurene begin post-op chemotherapy as soon as her wounds healed from the surgery.

Out of the Inferno

The doctor left us as the Houston skyline dimmed outside the hospital window. You could hear his rapid footsteps clacking on the polished floor die away. Down the hall, a patient called out for a nurse in a frantic tone, and the nurse answered from her station. You could hear evening news spilling out from the next room. Laurene sipped some water through a straw, and tears dropped from her face to her hospital gown. ***"RATS! RATS! RATS!"*** she said.

On the flight back to Grand Rapids, Laurene couldn't sit up, so she managed to lay across the window and middle seat to rest her head on my lap. We discussed how we would inform the girls. We talked about scheduling a fitting for a prosthetic breast. She felt off balance when she walked. She asked me if I was still okay with her not scheduling reconstructive surgery. I agreed. She had been through too much to undergo more pain and risk. When I happened to mention how angry I was at the doctor in Grand Rapids, she gave me a firm response. The first and last time we discussed the subject.

"I have no time for negative thoughts," she said. "I have to focus on the positive."

I decided not to mention another source of my anger. Laurene's surgeon had cut her breast tissue off and left an incision scar that meandered from her armpit to down across her chest in a jagged line that looked more like she had been sliced in a knife fight than through surgery. The scar looked careless to me. I had also been told that radiation burns were a thing of the past. Her chest glowed bright red. In addition, I experienced a raw atavistic feeling, like a roving savage had dragged my wife out of our cave home and mutilated her in front of me. I had failed to keep her safe. I could not have protected her against what is not protectable, but I still felt guilty and humiliated. I hated the surgeon for what she had done, even though she had done nothing wrong.

These and similar thought processes plagued me during my weaker moments over the next ten years. To what extent had the cancer been caused by inherited genes, by family and work stress, by growing up in an area ridden with carcinogens? To what extent were the missteps in Laurene's diagnosis and treatment the responsibility of others? To what extent was I responsible as her caregiver? And when we had successes like favorable lab reports, to what extent were those successes the result of good medicine or mere luck or the grace of God?

And thinking about my own behavior, to what extent was I using my wife's cancer as a scapegoat for my shortcomings as a husband, father, and businessman? I knew there were no clear answers to these useless questions, but I still aggravated myself with them. Rather than stop the thoughts, I let them carry on like a stranger talking to me nonstop in the dark, talking at length about subjects the stranger knew nothing about.

That summer, my work habits nose-dived. I began to daydream during business reviews. I had trouble containing my emotions. I lost my composure in an early morning meeting over a productivity issue in the factory. I had trouble listening to people. Self-discipline and job focus slipped. The tasks that I used to do easily and well, became difficult and slow.

I stopped working out at the athletic club at five in the morning. I no longer arrived among the first in the office at the beginning of the work day. I stopped planning ahead. Rather than trying to make things happen, I drifted through the day, and left earlier than normal. I no longer felt that I was carrying my weight on the executive team. For the first time in my career, I felt intensely incompetent and irresponsible. Like a fraud. The hamster wheel of my job still spun, but I had was merely riding, not running to make the wheel go around.

I questioned my decision, so many years earlier, to launch a business career. One night, a dream reflected my gloomy daytime attitude. I dreamed that I had died at work from a heart attack, and the company had carried me by forklift to behind the factory where they buried me in a company cemetery. The gravestones were arranged in the columns and rows of an organization chart. When I woke, the thought of having my identity defined in such a narrow way bothered me. The disruptive influence of a serious family illness was causing me to raise unwanted questions about the trajectory of my life. Was it time to edit my own narrative? For the time, I suppressed the idea. More than ever, we needed my executive pay and benefits. I also had four college educations to pay for. For a little longer, I retained the false belief that I was in charge.

Nothing seemed to help. Distracted from work, one moment I thought about how awful it would be to lose my wife, and what my life would be like without her. How could I navigate my life without Laurene? Would I stay single or remarry? Would I keep my job or do something else? Would I stay in Michigan, or move? In other moments, I engaged in fantasies about adventures to remote places, like taking a marine ferry to Alaska or hiking the Appalachian Trail. Or simply finding a golf instructor to teach me how to play a better game of golf, the biggest fantasy of all.

I acted on one of my wild ideas—ownership of a fancy sports car. I decided that my old, reliable Dodge Minivan was no longer a satisfying form of transportation. I bought a dark green Mitsubishi 3000 GT with a big engine, custom wheels, and fat tires. Laurene insisted that we buy the car on the last day of the month on the last day of the year to get the best deal. When she passed me in her Lexus on the way home from the dealership, I floored the accelerator and turned on the headlights. The headlight covers flipped up like Batman's armored, gadget-laden Bat mobile. We kept trading the lead as we circled Grand Rapids on I-96. We flashed our lights, waved playfully as we passed. I loved that little green sports car. I liked the way the wide tires held the road. I liked the way I had to drop down into the low seat. Driving the 3000 GT with abandon was my superficial attempt to get back in the driver's seat.

That summer, we decided to schedule a second opinion at The Cleveland Clinic. I remember sitting in the sparse waiting room in Cleveland. It seemed that most of the women sitting there that day were tall like Laurene. I wondered if tall women were more susceptible to breast cancer—maybe because of something related to their growth, or maybe because tall women had more cells? Idle thoughts.

After reviewing Laurene's records, the physician confirmed MD Anderson's diagnosis, adding that she had a 10% probability of surviving five years. It sounded like a death sentence (you have a ninety percent chance of being dead in five years). The statement turned out to be more precise than accurate. We drove back to Grand Rapids sobered by what we had heard. MD Anderson had refused to give us such specific information, even though we had asked. This was the first time we heard anyone characterize her prognosis as terminal. We had hoped that the Cleveland Clinic would see something more hopeful in her charts. As we passed the mile markers on the Ohio Turnpike back to Michigan, Laurene wondered out loud how a good God could give her such terrible news. She had already had her share of life's troubles. This was supposed to be a happy time.

Laurene never stopped trying to reconcile her belief in God with her grounded personality. In her mind, her successes in life had been driven more by hard work than as a result of faith and miracles. Her mantra had always been: *God helps those who help themselves.* Her statement that she needed to work hard on her faith demonstrated that the Christian belief of grace as the free and unmerited favor of God did not entirely comfort her. It was a passive concept. How could you *surrender to God, trust in the Lord, wait on the Lord?* She was more than willing to be generous and merciful to others, but she wanted to earn her own success and salvation. Her cancer was a problem to be solved, a disease to be controlled and beaten into submission like an unruly force of nature.

In September 1992, Laurene returned to Houston for post-op chemotherapy, a second round of the three-drug cocktail FAC (5-Fluorouracil, Adriamycin, Cyclophosphamide). She lost her hair a second time along with other common side effects like mouth sores, but she remained free of infections. We hoped that the second round would knock out the stubborn cancer. We wanted to believe that she had been cured. We evaluated whether or not to begin hormone therapy after the chemo. After our visit to the Cleveland Clinic, we were inclined to accept her doctor's the recommendation to begin taking Tamoxifin, an estrogen inhibitor that also prevented bone loss.

In addition to the seriousness of her prognosis, the main consideration had to do with Laurene's positive estrogen receptors (ER+). Tamoxifen had the potential to block the effects of estrogen on the growth of breast cancer cells, and to prevent the spread of cancer to other sites. We had concerns about some of the potential side effects: hot flashes, vaginal dryness, discharge or irritation, disinterest in sex, and we also had concerns about the increased risk of uterine cancer, ovarian cysts, and blood clots. Laurene decided to proceed, and she continued the hormone therapy for five years.

After almost a full year of treatment, we began the "new normal" phase of our cancer journey. Laurene set up a personal consulting company, and sub-contracted marketing research projects with a prestigious international consulting firm. Jennifer, Laurene's oldest, was getting good grades and her soccer team made the high school regional playoffs. Meredith surrounded herself with close friends, and performed well in middle school. Amy, my oldest, graduated from high school in Cleveland, and moved in with us to begin her freshman year at Kendall College of Art and Design. Laura, my youngest, was still in high school running relays on the track team, and checking out colleges. Except for the nagging fear of recurrence, and occasional checkups, we enjoyed day-to-day living. Laurene tolerated Tamoxifen without significant side effects. The intervals between check-ups at MD Anderson lengthened from three months to six months to annually. When we traveled to the Clinic for appointments, Laurene would say, "I'm going to get my good news today."

As for me, work never returned to normal. My performance continued to suffer. I had been like a working machine my whole career with no breaks between college, graduate school, and jobs. I had moved up the ladder on schedule—manager in my twenties, director in my thirties, vice president in my forties. But something had snapped like an overstretched rubber band. In addition to slacking off, I started making mistakes. The tight grip that I had held on my behavior and my work discipline loosened further. The changes in behavior may have been healthy, but in the business world, physical and mental health were trumped by things like attendance to detail, avoidance of surprises, and the production of results. My generation of business people had been raised on principals of tough-minded management, total dedication to the job, and loyalty to the organization.

I began to take more time off from work. After a full year of cancer treatment, Laurene wanted to travel. We visited England, Germany, Switzerland, Italy, Jerusalem, Cairo, Tokyo, Kyoto, Beijing, Hong Kong, Hawaii, Australia, and New Zealand. We pushed on with ambitious itineraries in spite of her discomfort and fatigue, an infection in Australia, stomach flu in Hawaii, and a broken arm in England. Even though were laid up for a week or so in hotels in a few places, we made the best of our temporary confinement. We rested and read books during the day, and managed to sample local food and entertainment. We were blessed with the services of excellent local physicians. I enjoyed a few diversions on my own: hiking in the English countryside, windsurfing off the rocky shoreline near Hilo, snorkeling at the Great Barrier Reef. When Laurene felt better, we resumed our travels.

We both experienced the best of life on the road. The green hills of the Cotwolds, Westminster Abbey, the small towns resting on the Lake of Constance, the flowered footbridges in Luzern, Michelangelo's Sistine Chapel ceiling, the fishing boats on the Sea of Galilee, the Temple Mount in Jerusalem, the Cairo Museum, the Summer Palace in Beijing, vessel-filled Victoria Harbor in Hong Kong, and the tea houses and temples of Kyoto. In contrast to our honeymoon, Laurene did the planning. We had a printed itinerary and a folder of confirmed reservations. Laurene didn't trust baggage handling, so we each carried our extra clothes in a small black roller bag.

A Husband's Passage Through Cancerland

Our three days in Kyoto remain my favorite memory of our travels. On the first day, we had been walking through the ancient city all morning, and wanted to find a place to sit and eat. We entered the grounds of a temple through a pathway lined by splashing fountains. We removed our shoes, and a silent attendant appeared in traditional dress. She guided us through bamboo curtains to a sparse but beautiful room with high ceilings and marble floors. In turns, she looked into our eyes and smiled deeply. Her thick, black hair gave off the luster of polished coal.

We sat down on tatami mats, and sipped ice cold water from small stone vessels. Chopsticks rested on smooth black stones. Fragrant tea arrived next which the attendant prepared with a bamboo whisk. Next, she disappeared and reappeared with a cup of briny broth, and side dishes served on lacquered trays. Without words or a menu, the shy attendant brought us condiments, sashimi, sushi, soba noodles, and quail eggs. She treated us with such gentleness and kindness and respect that we savored each long moment of our meal, trying to mimic her helpful gestures about how to pick up or stir our food. A presentation of sweets ended the meal.

Laurene and I were the only ones in the room. Other than our attendant, we didn't see another person. I felt transported to a holy place. A contentment settled over and around me in the soft light of the soft city. Laurene looked beautiful sitting across from me. She looked peaceful. In the temple, I felt like we had found a place suspended in time where no one worried, no one craved what they couldn't have, no one suffered pain or discomfort, and only good things happened. I completely forgot about our troubles.

Outside the temple, Laurene looked relieved to see that her shoes rested where she had left them. As she tied them on, her peaceful demeanor morphed back to tourist mode.

"This is a ***MUST DO*** experience for anyone visiting Kyoto. The food was great!"

"***MUST BE*** experience" I replied. The quiet surroundings, not the food, had been the highlight for me.

"Very funny," Laurene said, half-ignoring me while she examined a Kyoto street map. "Let's see where we can go next. We need more gifts."

Now it was time to shop for the girls, an activity just as life-affirming and sacred to Laurene as the quiet lunch had been for me. On our way out of the temple, she spied a porcelain-faced woman in Geisha attire passing slowly by in the back of a long limousine. The Geisha and Laurene exchanged looks, and Laurene motioned to her with her ever-present camera. The woman asked the uniformed driver to stop. She rolled down the window so Laurene could take snapshots. Laurene felt triumphant! She had captured another special moment.

LESSON FIVE

We open our eyes to sacred sparks in everyday life. What sparks one person goes unnoticed by another. The bouncing, dark eyes of the Geisha woman in a black limo sparked Laurene. The candles, incense, and trickling water of a Buddhist temple enlivened the sacred in me.

6.

*"...Arrogance, greed, and envy—those are
 the three switches
That start people's hearts." Then he fell silent.
I said, "You'd be doing me a favor if you'd go on
 talking.
So I can make some sense of this.*

Dante's Inferno, Canto VI

One winter morning in 1996, Haworth asked me to leave the company.

They had tolerated the ups and downs of my performance long enough. What would I tell Laurene? She had never been fired. What would I tell my dad and my father-in-law? Dad had never been fired. Neil had never been fired. After military service in WWII, they had each been employed by the same employer from their first until their last day of work. They had retired with pensions and benefits. I had worked since fourteen without losing a job. While I felt sorry for people when they were laid off or removed for any reason, I had the arrogance to think that nothing like this would ever happen to me.

At age forty-nine, I was on the street for the first time. Three of our four daughters were in college. I had tuition, room, and board to pay, not to mention sorority dues, junior year abroad, and other expenses. I lived in a large house with a big mortgage in a fancy neighborhood. We belonged to an athletic club and a country club. Haworth had paid me well, along with automotive, executive health, and financial planning allowances. Every morning, I had pulled my car into my own covered parking space—a "man in full" about to be consumed by "the bonfire of the vanities," as Tom Wolfe would say.

I called Laurene. I gave no excuses. Laurene asked me questions about my separation agreement. She didn't blame me or panic. She simply wanted to help me find a new job. She also said that she would find a way to work again. A few weeks later, she landed a job teaching marketing at a local college. When I called Dad, he gave me a pep talk, but also expressed concern that I had already worked ten years each for two employers. I knew what he thought: even though I had only worked for three employers in nearly 30 years, he worried that I would be tagged as a job hopper. He still lived in the fast-vanishing world of lifetime employment. Neil never said a word, but I knew he hoped that this change might land us closer to Texas.

I set up office in an outplacement firm paid for by Haworth. I looked at job opportunities throughout the United States, but I paid special attention to openings in Houston. Moving to Houston would place us near MD Anderson, and also near Neil and Stella.

A ten-minute commute, Laurene and I had lunch almost every day at home (eating out had all but disappeared, since Laurene had taken an ax to our family budget). She helped me throughout my job research. She supported me in every way she could, and although I knew she was anxious about the loss of income, she never complained or pressured me. I worked hard on my search, and after a few weeks, I was given a key to the office so I could get in before regular hours. I was soon scheduling job interviews in New York, Chicago, San Francisco, Minneapolis, Portland, Oregon—and Houston!

When I returned from an interview in Houston, I expected Laurene to be ecstatic.

If I received a job offer, we could move to her hometown and spend more time with her parents. She could be close to MD Anderson for her cancer check-ups. Since only Meredith still lived at home, we would only have one daughter to relocate. I would be elected an officer of a computer manufacturer ten times larger than Haworth: Compaq Computer Corporation. No matter the location, this was a huge step up in my career. I had always been envious of the high tech industry. It seemed more exciting than mainstream manufacturing.

Rather than say how nice or what wonderful news, Laurene posed her inimitable questions while I

Out of the Inferno

stood in front of her wearing a golf hat embroidered with a red Compaq logo:

"Where did you get the hat?"

"They have a logo store where you can buy hats and shirts and all kinds of neat stuff." I showed her two logoed golf shoe bags. "I bet you didn't know this, I sure didn't—Compaq sponsors the David Pelz World Putting Championship!"

"So that impresses you...," Laurene said. I could see this conversation was about to take a turn for the worse.

"More important...the stock is going up like a rocket," I said. I thought that she would be impressed with the stock performance, if not the cool swag. I began to place the the Compaq merchandise back into a white plastic bag printed with another red Compaq logo.

"Nice...when you're done showing me all this free stuff, you may want to hear about a little research I did on Compaq." Rather than looking me in the eye, she looked down at her notes.

"What did you find?"

"The company's walking in tall grass right now, but management over-reports sales by shipping computers from the factory to company-owned warehouses, and by stuffing their dealer distribution channels with unsold product to meet quarterly sales targets. That's misleading to investors, and not acceptable accounting practice."

"Didn't your company used to do that?"

"GE still breaks accounting rules. That doesn't make it right."

"What else did you find?"

"The top dogs are having extra-marital affairs."

"How in the world do you know that?"

"Photos on the society page of the *Houston Chronicle*—the Chairman takes his mistress to charity events—lucky for him he's not married to a Texan."

"Why?"

"Because he'd be dead."

"So you'd shoot *me* if I had an affair."

"*Guaranteed.* In Texas, shooting your spouse for screwing around gets you punished about the same as running a stop sign."

"Now hold on just a minute, Laurene. This is a big company, and they like me. And besides, the man I would work for went on and on about his family."

"I know about him. He's a nice family man, but did you know he plans to retire by the end of the year?"

"Laurene, how do you know that?"

"I have lots of friends in Houston."

"He'll be replaced with someone decent."

"A fish rots from the head," she replied. "It will do no good to move to Houston, if the company isn't right. You can wear your fancy new hat on your way to the unemployment office."

"Have you read their mission—?"

"—mission statements are crap."

"Laurene."

"Sugar Bear, you need to be less trusting."

"So you're against this?"

"Your decision. I've said all I'm going to say."

And just like her father, she kept her word. She never mentioned the subject again.

Laurene said all of this in a firm but quiet tone. She had a way of talking with people in general, but especially with people she loved, that didn't place you on the defensive. Her line of reasoning was logical, but not judgmental.

Six months after my last day at Haworth, I received the offer from Compaq, and accepted—more pay, stock options, a brand new company laptop, and lots of logo wear. Meredith, didn't want to leave her friends in Grand Rapids, but she was a trooper like her mother. She tested and interviewed at the John Cooper School, a private, college prep school in The Woodlands, a suburb near my new office. We rented an apartment so Meredith could attend the first day of class in August 1996.

When Meredith arrived in Houston, Neil took her out to buy school clothes. "I guess you feel you've ruined your life by moving to Texas, but you saved mine. I owe you." Neil took her to the same place where he had purchased school clothes for Laurene—a Sears store near their neighborhood.

On my first day of work at Compaq, I attended the Monday morning staff meeting, and sat beside my new boss who, just as Laurene had predicted announced his retirement. He introduced me to the rest of his staff. Near the end of the meeting, the annual United Way Campaign kicked off with a heart-tugging video. Tears formed in my eyes, and began to roll down my cheeks before I could catch them. My boss said, "My God, what have we done!" Later the controller told me that his eyes hadn't been dry either.

Unfortunately, the same controller dropped into my office a few months later, crying about more than a United Way video. Believe me, you don't ever want to see an accountant cry. He informed me that Compaq had been inflating sales in the way Laurene had described, and that the practice was driven by top management. Consistent with the corporate mission statement, the controller wanted my help in exercising his right to appeal unethical and legal conduct. Shortly after I initiated the appeal on his behalf, I received a call from a senior officer at the head office. He informed me that I needn't get involved with the appeal, because the concern would be addressed at the corporate level.

Compaq was at the height of corporate success in 1996 with record sales and profits that increased its cash from $700 million to nearly $5 billion. Other than IBM, Compaq had outdistanced its PC competitors and was driving some of them out of the market. Gateway Computers, in particular, was imploding, and Compaq filling their market space. To support the rapid increase in business, I hired ten contract recruiters to supplement my fulltime staffing department. In North America, we hired 150 professionals a month—product marketers, design engineers, technical reps, customer service people. I had never been busier in my life, but it was great fun while it lasted, and the man who replaced my retiring boss, really was a family man and a supremely astute computer tech executive.

Shortly after we arrived in Houston, Laurene and I began house hunting. Laurene invited John, her ex-husband, to join us. He worked in Houston as a radiation physicist at MD Anderson (over the next ten years, John would quietly oversee his ex-wife's radiation treatments). Even though they were divorced, I could tell that Laurene still loved him. She had a heart like a steel trap, and once she had let someone into her life, she wouldn't let go. We would enter the door of a prospective house, and Laurene would introduce us to the real estate agent as Randy, my husband, and John, my ex-husband. John and I were about the same height, with thick brown hair and wire glasses. You can imagine the stares. John and I thought the situation was hilarious. Later, Laurene said to me, "John has a good mind, and we can use his advice."

After our second counter offer had been accepted, Laurene sat alone in the house for an hour to make think about the deal. The lower floor contained a master bedroom suite, formal living and dining rooms, and a guest bedroom. The second floor comprised an additional three bedrooms and an upstairs family room. The backyard was wild with overgrowth, but within a year, Laurene landscaped the year, and designed a pool with fountains and brickwork to match the house. An eight-foot high wooden fence surrounded the property. On day, I called one of the pool contractors to complain, because he had yelled at Laurene. She felt that her concern had been dismissed, and that she had been talked down to because she was a woman. "I don't care if she's a squirrel," the contractor said, "that woman's difficult to please."

In 1998, Compaq acquired Digital Equipment Corporation for $9 billion, an industry record. Digital employed twice as many people as Compaq, but with only half of Compaq's revenue. By this time, I had been elected by Compaq's Board to Vice President, Human Resources, Quality and Customer Service for Compaq's worldwide sales, marketing, and service organizations. My job was to recommend a North American integration strategy for the two companies for sales, marketing, and customer service. I managed an integration team with representatives from both companies, along with the support of twenty McKinsey consultants.

I conducted integration meetings in Boston, Hong Kong, Singapore, and Japan. I slept on airplanes rather than hotel rooms, and when in Houston, sometimes passed the night on the floor of my office.

The integration teams of operating people from Digital and Compaq, recommended that the new company be staffed from a customer perspective, in other words, from the bottom up. The senior McKinsey people disagreed. They developed a plan to staff from the top down with alternating layers of Digital and Compaq executives leading functional departments. The consultants won the day. My job was offered to my counterpart at Digital. Over 2,000 Compaq employees and 15,000 Digital employees were laid off. I was one of them. Now, I really did feel like a job hopper.

So less than two years after moving to Houston, I once again set up office in an outplacement agency to look for work. As it turns out, I left at the right time. Compaq's continued management misconduct, along with the incompatibility of the Compaq and Digital cultures, led to a permanent downward spiral resulting the demise of the Chairman and the rest of the Board. The best operating executives left ahead of the fiasco, including Tim Cook, who later succeeded Steve Jobs at the top of Apple Computer. Today, the ex-Compaq Linked-in group reads like a "Who's Who" in the American technology industry.

Compaq's stock plummeted to less than half of what it had been when I worked for the company, and in 2002, Compaq signed a $25 billion merger agreement with Hewlett-Packard. Today, the remains of the largest PC company of the 1990s can be found

Out of the Inferno

in some of HP's low-end systems products. A significant portion of the beautiful campus where I interviewed for my job, including two eight-story reinforced concrete buildings, fell to a planned implosion in 2011. Every member of Compaq's senior management save one was let go shortly after I left. The 1991 Harvard Business School Case Study about Compaq's remarkable success was revised in 2003, and titled "Compaq's Struggle," a euphemism for what actually happened.

Laurene never said I told you so. If corporations are "persons" in the eyes of the law, Compaq died of internal injuries. The Chairman was fired, but to my knowledge, he was never shot by his wife.

***

Laurene continued to be healthy. She had five years of "all clear" checkups behind her, but the threat of a recurrence continued to haunt us. Even though it would have been convenient to stay in Houston, Laurene encouraged me to find the next best job for my career anywhere in the United States, as she had when I left Haworth. Initially, I focused my search in Houston, but other than consulting work, nothing turned up. After the intensity of my Compaq experience, I felt burnt out. My stomach hurt most of the time. Also, I didn't have the same focus on finding another job as I had when I left Haworth. My career orientation that had lessened during my waning days at Haworth seemed to be falling away altogether. For the first time in my life, I became more reflective about my life work. I had done well, but at what price? What had I sacrificed? Now I questioned how I wanted to spend the rest of my life.

Laurene and I talked about how our career aspirations had changed over our lives. She had wanted to become a lawyer, but her parents had discouraged her at a time when teaching and nursing were sanctioned as the most appropriate female occupations. She majored in political science at Sam Houston State to keep her hopes alive, but settled for a teaching certificate and later a graduate degree in education from the University of Texas. Single motherhood had driven her into the MBA Program at Case Western University in her late thirties. She needed to support her children. In my case, I had started a business career the day after I graduated from college as an English major. I had worked straight for twenty-eight years, except for an educational leave to earn an MBA from Columbia University. We had both been driven by economic considerations more than anything. Now that our "big three" daughters were nearly through college, what would we do next?

During the two years I had worked at Compaq, Laurene reconnected with all of her Texas friends from grade school through college. She attended all the Compaq spouse events. We continued to travel on my vacations. On Saturday nights, we went out to dinner, and then stopped to visit Neil and Stella on our way home. We usually found them sitting in the recreation room watching John Wayne movies.

Laurene spent a good deal of her free time focusing on her parents, taking them to doctor's appointments, running errands for them, helping them stay in touch with their friends. She waned to take care of them as they had done for her. One day Laurene took Neil to a video store to help him sign up for a membership, because Laurene knew he loved to watch Westerns. She had purchased a video player for her parents for Christmas. Neil and Stella looked at the black box on top of the TV like an alien object from outer space had landed in their house. Laurene gave up after Neil refused to show the video store manager his driver's license. "That's kind of personal," he said.

Neil and Stella's health continued on a downward spiral. Neil had heart disease and bladder cancer, and Stella became increasingly disabled from rheumatoid arthritis, a condition that affected her heart as well. Both died while we were in Houston. We were with each of them until the end, a blessing for having moved to Houston. Whenever they were in the hospital, Laurene refused to leave their sides overnight, unless someone else from the family stayed with them—another one of her rules. We all took our turns. The last time I sat with Neil, he surprised me by kissing me on the lips, uncommon for a man from central Texas. He passed away on February 5, 1997. At the cemetery, two overweight Marines played scratchy Taps on a cassette player, and presented Stella with a neatly folded American flag. Stella followed the next year, July 9, 1998, succumbing to numerous strokes and her arthritis. "We partied so hard our whole lives, it's no wonder we both pooped out," she said.

As the only child of Neil and Stella, Laurene deeply mourned the loss of her parents. Their deaths brought her own thoughts of death closer. She wanted the best good-bye ceremonies for Neil and Stella. At Stella's viewing, someone had smeared bright red lipstick on Stella's mouth. As she lay in her open casket, the lipstick made her look clownish. Laurene raised cane until the funeral director fixed her mother's face. Over the next few years, Laurene cared for Neil and Stella's aging friends and relatives. We visited them in their homes and in the hospital, attended church with them, and sat through their funerals. We loved to hear people tell stories about her parents. The girls and I joined her in these visits all over Texas. "Your roots," Laurene would say.

Laurene commented on death in the world around her—in a bird that lay dead outside our kitchen window, in the tragic death of Princess Diana, in the old people at her parents' funerals, in anything swept away in the rain. She wanted to talk about the routines of dying—hospital, hospice, viewings, memorial services, and burials. She commented on how church women prepared finger sandwiches, potato salad, punch, and cookies in the church basement. We talked about how we had missed contacting a few people when her parents had died, and the need to get her address book up to date. The plusses and minuses of funerals vs. memorial services, open vs. closed casket viewings, how to instruct florists and plan the music. She seemed to be rehearsing.

LESSON SIX

When someone who loves you says that you're about to do something stupid…listen.

7.

*We made our way down to the fourth concavity
along the sad-making embankment…
Watching this, I felt heartbroken….*

Dante's Inferno, Canto VII

The veil had not yet closed over Compaq, so I was a red hot commodity in the high tech arena. On November 1, 1998, I joined Intuit, Inc., a financial and tax preparation software company in the San Francisco Bay Area, as VP Human Resources. When I informed the company that Laurene would stay in Houston until Meredith graduated from high school, my boss worked out an arrangement for me to fly home every other Wednesday for a long weekend. Alternatively, if Laurene could fly out to San Francisco, they would pay for her flight. I called Laurene in Houston after my first day on the new job.

"How was your first day at work?"

"Fun but weird. A young product manager was having a one-on-one meeting with her boss. He wasn't listening to her. He kept taking long phone calls. She decided to get his attention by taking her blouse off."

"What did the boss do?"

"He ran out of the office screaming for his secretary to call HR. Now my staff wants me to tell them what to do."

"Your staff should be able to handle something like this. They're testing you."

"Do you think so?"

"I've told you before, you're naive. People take advantage of you."

"If you had taken your blouse off at General Electric, what would they have done?"

"I would have never done that."

"This is a hypothetical question. What would GE have done?"

"Fired me."

"Well, I think a written warning might be the answer."

When I recommended a written warning, everyone thought this action was way too harsh. Besides, the boss had not been listening. After much discussion, the company provided the woman with a personal coach, and the manager was shipped off for training to improve his active listening skills.

I loved living in the Bay Area. I began to relax. I daydreamed about developing a hobby. I stopped reading only business books, and began to read for enjoyment. Laurene loved to hear me tell stories about my new work culture. She flew out to attend some of the employee meetings and parties. We also explored the coast from the Monterrey Peninsula to Napa Valley and Santa Rosa. On one of her trips, we purchased and began to furnish a three-story townhouse in Los Gatos, a beautiful small town in the foothills of the Santa Cruz Mountains. The stucco townhouse sat against a steep hill with a pergola on one side, a five-minute walk from the center of town. Every week night I took long walks after dinner. I remember looking with envy through restaurant windows at couples laughing and talking while they drank wine and ate dinner. I wanted to move Laurene out to California as soon as she was free. I missed her.

On the weekends when I stayed in the Bay Area, I often drove over the mountains to Santa Cruz, one of the most beautiful places on earth. I walked along the pier or sat on the beach. I took a group fishing charter, and caught rock bass. I rode the train from Palo Alto into San Francisco to see the museums, and walk around Union Square. On another weekend, I drove to Sausalito for lunch where I bought a copper water fountain for my office (everyone at Intuit seemed to have little fountains in their offices). I purchased a mountain bike, and explored the bike trails around Los Gatos, stopping for a latte afterwards. The alternating weekends in Houston gave us time to take trips to the Hill Country, and enjoy Meredith's senior year in high school. We talked about our future as empty nesters.

On one of my solo weekends, I decided to go camping at one of the many beautiful state parks that dot the California Coast. I had ordered an Alaskan Guide Tent from LL Bean, a purchase Laurene would have never approved. When I tried to pitch the enormous tent in sandy beach grass, it ballooned in the heavy sea breeze like an out-of-control parachute. After amusing two children at the next campsite for fifteen minutes, they came over to help me stake the green monster down.

I set up a cot inside, then went to a hot dog stand on the beach for supper. That night, I fell into the deepest sleep I can remember. When I woke up in the morning, I felt like a new person. I lit a small fire, and fried bacon and scrambled eggs in a small cast iron skillet. I perked coffee over the campfire. I sat in a canvas chair for two hours drinking coffee, watching all the activity in the campground, and not thinking about a thing. I spent the entire day sitting and walking around the shore. The sea tide and the cloudless sky calmed me.

The time I spent on my new job in California gave me a needed break from the weight of worry about Laurene. For all we knew she had been cured.

A Husband's Passage Through Cancerland

And I was also relieved to be out of the pressure-cooker environment at Compaq, lucky to be working in a people-friendly work culture. I've heard lots of complaints about California, mostly from those who have never lived there. There was a gentleness in how people related to each other. Drivers actually stopped at crosswalks, and I seldom heard honking horns. Street people didn't worry about freezing to death overnight. I could order a whole milk mocha topped with whipped cream from a vegan barista without a judging stare. I might have stayed for the rest of my career or the rest of my life. California turned out to be a healing place.

The new work culture started to influence me. A few months after I began my employment at Intuit, a director who reported to me asked for a six-month leave of absence. He told me that he felt like a large curtain had fallen on him, and he had to get "right with Buddha" before he could be effective at work. At the moment, his rationale shocked me, but I signed the approvals for an unpaid leave. That weekend, I drove over to Santa Cruz and sat on the beach. I purchased a cup of clam chowder, and a carton of bay shrimp for lunch. I thought about what my director had said in a different light. What if not being "right with God" disabled me from doing my work? How much more important would faith be in my life, if I depended on faith to guide me every hour of every day?

Out of the Inferno

I decided to call the director to see how his spiritual work was going on the cliffs of the Big Sur. He told me that at the moment he was resting naked on an outdoor massage table doing bodywork with a topless masseuse. "Incredible," he said. "You should come down here for a weekend workshop." When I mentioned that Intuit intended to acquire a new company and I could use his help, he promised to call me back in a month or so. I had to perform the acquisition due diligence myself. The relationship between bodywork and enlightenment escaped me. Perhaps too much sitting meditation had stiffened his muscles? Perhaps Laurene was right when she said, "I've told you before...you're naive."

In April 1999, Laurene traveled with Laura to London and Paris. She wanted to develop a closer relationship with her stepdaughter. Beyond the cities, they also visited neighboring towns and the countryside. The pictures from the trip included a snapshot of Laura sitting among pink-and-white tulips in Claude Monet's garden at Giverny. The two had a great time together, and a special bond formed. Laurene's idea for the trip also resulted out of her sense of fairness. Amy had studied at the Royal College of Art in London during her junior year at Kendall College.

I had worked at Intuit for almost a year. I liked the people, and I liked the work. I looked forward to the youngest of our four daughters setting off for college. Meredith had excelled academically at the John Cooper School, and had run low hurdles on the track team. She applied to and received acceptance at Vanderbilt University in Nashville. Once Meredith started college, our commuter marriage would end. Everything seemed to be coming together. We would sell the house in Houston, and Laurene would join me in Los Gatos for life in a new and fascinating part of the country. I would no longer have to spend my work evenings alone. Laurene talked about going back to work or involving herself in the community.

In May, I had just returned to the Bay Area after celebrating Mother's Day in Houston. I was in my office sipping coffee while pouring over documents for a new business plan. Laurene and I normally talked on the telephone once or twice a day, often in the morning before work or late in the evening. Receiving a phone call from her during working hours surprised me.

"The cancer's come back," she said in a quiet voice.

"I'll fly home today," I said.

"I'm sorry."

I looked out my office window searching for anything ordinary. A car pulled out of the parking lot, a jet flew overhead towards a landing in San Mateo, the tops of two sails appeared on the small lake beyond the office complex. I heard people chatting outside my office. I wanted to see or hear any signs of normal life to offset hearing my wife apologize for something she had no part in causing. I don't remember anything else she said, but it was a short conversation. I sobbed after the call ended. My body shook like a personal earthquake.

I cancelled meetings, and took the next available flight home. I felt suspended during the flight. I couldn't talk to anyone or do anything. To be inert at 30,000 feet in the middle of a crisis felt like torture. Worst case scenarios spun though my mind like spasms. I had recently re-organized my life. Now everything was once again up in the air—the uncertain air. I felt a general feeling of disorder, unsettledness—again. Laurene's bones were now occupied with metastatic cancer like dandelions that had popped up overnight on a perfectly green lawn. How could we get those cells (a million or a billion of them?) out of her body, starve them or asphyxiate them? Would Laurene ever feel well again? What would happen to our happy thoughts about the future? What about my job?

All the way home, I kept thinking about the decision we had made a year earlier to stop the Tamoxifen. Research had indicated no change in survivorship for postmenopausal women after five years of the hormone treatment. Now after six years, bony metastases had been identified through a routine bone scan. When Laurene said that the cancer had come back, I think she meant that cancer had re-entered our lives in a big new way. Although the term is used loosely, "recurrence" most often refers to another cancer in the primary site of origin (where the cancer started), the same breast or in lymph nodes nearby. Cancer cells that travel to a distant site, in this case, Laurene's bones, are more accurately termed metastatic cancer, a condition far more serious than a local recurrence. (Tumors caused by the cells that have spread are called secondary tumors.) I think people may prefer "recurrence," because the word sounds less sinister than "metastasis."

We had been concerned about the side effects of Tamoxifin: increased risk of cancer of the uterus, strokes, and clots in the lungs. I remembered the warning following the long list of negative potential outcomes. "If you are thinking about taking Tamoxifen to reduce the chance that you will develop breast cancer, you should talk to your doctor about the risks and benefits of this treatment." We had followed the best available advice. The cancer had spread. I had little problem making business decisions with imperfect information, but life and death decisions bothered me. We would have to live with the consequences. Second guessing had little value.

The following week, Laurene resumed taking Tamoxifin. Since the cancer had not entered the soft tissues (liver, lungs), we hoped that the hormone therapy would contain the cancer or make it go away. When we revisited the library to view the latest research, we found that the survival odds were not good—the average life expectancy with metastatic breast cancer was 27 months. We had always ignored the odds in the past. Laurene had already survived beyond the Cleveland Clinic's dire prediction that she had a 10% chance of surviving five years. Laurene had now survived eight years to the month after she first felt an abnormality in her breast. Other than occasional fatigue, she felt fine. She wanted to travel. The balance of 1999 would be a year to celebrate life. Laurene informed the girls that new "unexpected challenges" awaited us.

We decided that her two girls had to go to Europe next. In July, Jennifer, Meredith, Laurene and I traveled to southern Germany. We stayed in a hotel in Stein am Rhein, a beautiful walled town where the Bodensee ("sea at the bottom") and the Rhein River converge. We walked back and forth on the footbridge to Switzerland, visited some business friends, then drove down to Luzern. We were following about the same itinerary as we had during our haphazard honeymoon twelve years earlier—southern Germany, Switzerland, and Italy. Meredith had dated a Swiss exchange student named Marco during her senior year, so we spent several days with his family in Brig near Geneva. We witnessed Marco undergoing his physical for the Swiss Army in the town square along with the other eighteen-year-olds, and took day trips to Lake Geneva and Zermatt. After leaving Marco's family, we drove through the Simplon Pass into Italy to visit Lucca, Portofino, Pisa, Siena, Florence, Venice, and Milan. Laurene wanted to see everything. She wore us out! Our days were so filled, we often missed meals, something you should never allow in Italy.

In addition to the Tamoxifen, Laurene began a series of hormone therapy treatments (oral bisphosphonates) to slow the bone damage and reduce the risk of fractures. The treatments were accompanied by fatigue, anemia, nausea, extreme bone and joint pain. Friends and family drove Laurene down to the clinic so I could continue working at Intuit. The treatments didn't have any effect, so towards the end of the year, Laurene began an experimental Taxol chemotherapy program. The program also required weekly treatments, so beginning November 1, Intuit granted me Family Medical Leave that would run through February 2000. Laptops weren't as functional as they are these days, but I could get some work done from home or by sitting beside Laurene's bed at the clinic while she received her infusions. I was beginning to think it would be impossible to return to Intuit after my leave. In her Christmas letter that year, Laurene wrote lovingly that I had become her "chauffeur, personal shopper, chef, and nurse."

Out of the Inferno

One afternoon back in Houston, I experienced a personal crisis. Laurene had sent me on an errand. I stood in the shopping hubbub of the Galleria, a fancy Houston shopping mall. I had stopped walking, because I suddenly felt confused and a bit dizzy. I felt caught up in an alien world. I was on a level halfway up overlooking the open mall, a blurry space between the artificial interior light of the mall and the natural light that filtered down from a large skylight. I could see the white ice of the skating rink below me, and feel the hot sun radiating through the glass roof above me.

I was overwhelmed by disorganized thoughts: *What was I doing outside the office in the middle of the day? I'm a businessman. My career has been cut off. My life has been muddled. I want to go back to work. I have more to do. I'm too young to retire. I don't want to be here. I'm useless. Would I be a coward to go back to work? Would I be a coward not to go back to work?*

I'm not sure how long I remained in this liminal space between everyday consciousness and a dream world. I felt like I had been transported into some kind of ancient ritual. The open floors and escalators displayed large and small people moving along the levels, up and down the atrium filled with artificial plants and trees. They looked like figures from another world. Had Dante been present, he could have descended from the daylight of the outer world to the lowest circle of hell to see the "emperor of the kingdom of woe" encased in a block of ice at the bottom while children skated in an oval rink. I stood in limbo like one of Dante's broken souls. I remained still and unmoving. The windup key that had kept me going, stuck, unmovable, in the middle of my back.

I continued gazing down at the children skating across the ice on the rink below. People sat nearby sipping Starbucks, as others passed me by on their way up or down the shopping levels. It was a Wednesday at three o'clock in the afternoon on an ordinary day, but I felt exposed, naked—like an embarrassed teenager with an invisible audience. Were people staring at me? My career plans, my grand schemes, the future of my life, my security and natural optimism had disintegrated. I stood blown clear of what I knew of life, and how I set myself apart from everyone else. This gap would play hell with my neat resume.

As my assistant at work would often say, "Sorry, he's out of the office today." This day, I *was* out of the office. My predictable sense of self had abandoned me to take the afternoon off. My usual way of being had taken a walk, and left whatever was left of me behind. My expensive suits, cufflink shirts, and flashy ties could no longer armor me against what my world had become. I felt like my clothes had turned wrong side out, and then disappeared.

Out of the Inferno

I honestly can't report precisely what happened at that moment or exactly how I felt, but I do know that what I experienced felt real to me. Two people passing by broke the spell.

A white-haired old man walked briskly by dragging a buxom young blond while she tripped forward to keep up in her high heels. All boobs and legs, she wore a precarious tank top and the shortest skirt I had ever seen. She whined wildly as she tripped forward, but the old man looked straight ahead while pulling her long thin arm like a rope. A black woman sitting beside me on a bench observed the couple, too. We turned our heads towards each other making eye contact with bemused smiles of some unspoken agreement between us. I felt a glimpse of the black woman's soul through her eyes. Maybe we both needed a break from what was foremost in our lives. We didn't speak to each other, but we shared this brief human comedy, or perhaps tragedy.

When I looked away, I felt like a spell had broken. I had a fresh air feeling in my chest. I don't know if the feeling came from the power of a divine intervention, or from the humorous experience I shared with the black woman, or watching the old geezer drag the long-legged girl though the mall. But at that point, I felt crystal clear about what to do next. I had a new occupation: caregiver.

LESSON SEVEN

If you are a woman, caregiving is the womanliest things you can do. If you are a man, it is one of the manliest things you can do.

8.

*And I'm abandoned; I sit and watch while Yes
And No (I will survive, I won't) wage war inside
my head.*

Dante's Inferno, Canto VIII

"What would you tell me to do if I was your wife?" Laurene asked her doctor.

"You're making an assumption that I love my wife," he chuckled.

Then he gave her his best advice, and finished by saying, "Twenty years from now, people will look back, and call people like me witch doctors. There is so much about cancer we don't know. Someday, cancer will be treated like a chronic disease. Fewer people will die of cancer, but we're not there yet." What he said made sense to me. Medicine is art more than science, and an imperfect art at best. From that day, Laurene referred to her oncologist as "my charming witch doctor."

At the end of an appointment, I asked Laurene's doctor about his worldwide reputation as an oncologist. "I have good hands," he said. With all the medical technology available to him, he still relied on his sense of touch. His hands could find tumors better than machines. During our office visits, he always asked Laurene to go first with her questions, but while she talked, his eyes began the examination, and his hands felt for physical evidence of what was going on in her body. He knew where he could press hard, and where he couldn't. Or he might warn her if his examination might cause her pain.

I believe that his healing touch and his healing words extended my wife's survival. He was one reason Laurene kept beating the odds, sitting on the tail end of the survival curve. He was also one of the humblest physicians I had ever met. Cancer humbles the most brilliant people. His caring, respectful doctor and patient relationship with Laurene would prove to be the most important relationship over the following ten years, second only to our relationship as man and wife.

Laurene liked the witch doctor term, because her perspective of medical care included the natural patterns of interpersonal caring, almost what shamans and other folk healers had provided before modern medicine. Her concept of caring did not include soothing statements or platitudes about healing, and certainly not unwanted hugs that would hurt her body. She wanted relationships with all of her caregivers, including me, that produced results—a warm blanket when she was chilled, remedies for extreme pain, facts and data about her disease, and support for her continuing right to find ways to survive.

A Husband's Passage Through Cancerland

My new job as a caregiver followed this pattern. Laurene's relationships with others confirmed the instrumental support I had given her so far. She might share more of her emotional needs with me later on, but for most of the years of her survival, improving the quality of her daily life was the gift I could give her. In many ways, my job description was not unlike tapping the strengths that I had used to make a living: showing up and getting things done. Maybe at some level, Laurene knew that this was all that I could do, and she didn't ask me for more. I don't know. I kept looking for ways to be useful. I bought her fresh flowers every week, and found other little things to please her, like baking her favorite toffee cookies from brown sugar and chopped Heath Bars.

Beyond the medical professionals at MD Anderson, Laurene received lots of "free" advice, all with good intentions, but not always helpful:

"You don't *look* like you have cancer."
"Maybe you don't have cancer."
"Turn everything over to the Lord."
"Why haven't you had surgery yet?"
"My grandmother died of breast cancer, but she was in her eighties."
"You're too young to have cancer."
"You can get through this. I know you."
"Have you tried flaxseed oil?"
"You need acupuncture."

Others stayed away from Laurene as if they might "catch" cancer from her. The truth is that cancer frightens people. They think, *"This could happen to me."* And it does. While we lived in Houston, two of Laurene's girlfriends were diagnosed with breast cancer, and one died. Some didn't want to be around a cancer patient because of their associations of cancer and death, and unmentionable subjects such as diarrhea, constipation, vomiting, and bleeding. Our Latina housekeeper told me, "My people think of cancer like the dirty laundry you keep hidden in your house."

Some people projected their own issues onto Laurene:

"When I told my husband I had cancer, he said he'd miss my cooking and then he left town."
"I hate mammograms. I need to get one. I would be so ashamed if I were diagnosed."
"Exercise. I need to get more exercise."
"I have good genes. No one in my family has ever had cancer."

A host of recommendations for alternative and complementary cancer therapies and treatments followed Laurene's recurrence: music, meditation, faith healing, massage, reflexology, chemicals and herbs, diets and exercise regimens, colon cleansing and chiropractors. When Laurene asked her doctor about these methods, she expected him to downplay their importance. Instead, his answer was so helpful that I have never forgotten what he said. "Some of these methods can relieve symptoms, ease side effects, or improve your quality of life. I only have one problem with alternative treatments. People feel like failures if they don't work."

So what helped? Friendships and her family sustained Laurene more than anything. Daily phone calls with Jennifer and Meredith, less frequent but important calls with Amy and Laura, and conversations with best friends helped. Laurene and I would always talk afterwards about what everyone had to say. These conversations kept her going and engaged in life. Sometimes she would talk for as much as an hour on one call, and then take a nap afterwards. I spent hours nearby listening to the soft cadence of her central Texas accent. Friendships built over her lifetime were far more important to her than anything. Laurene also surrounded her with a helping community of neighbors, church members, personal service providers, and counselors. She never turned anyone away who wanted to help, even people who were not helpful.

This support was not available to everyone we encountered. During the years of sitting in the waiting rooms of the clinic, in addition to words of hope, I overheard many sad conversations about people who were missing supportive friendships, as well as the family, community, and financial support to cope with their disease. Women would fail to make appointments, because they had no one to drive them. I heard stories about how patients had been abandoned by their husbands, separated or divorced, or by partners who disappeared when things got rough. I listened to single mothers tell how there was no one to care for their children during treatment. I overheard a mother and daughter arguing in hateful tones about whether or not the mother should check off "anger" as a concern on a survey form. *"I'M NOT ANGRY. DO YOU THINK I'M ANGRY?"* she yelled.

Costs and losses piled up on women with no one to help out. No one to translate. No one to take notes. No one to read instructions for medical regimens. No one to fill prescriptions. No one to help clean the house and do laundry when they hurt too much to move. Health insurance was another big issue. One black woman said her doctor told her to get a job with benefits before he would treat her. A Latina woman talked with a social worker about how she could qualify for a clinical trial—the woman could not speak English and she was an illegal immigrant. I heard so many conversations of oppression and social injustice. Sitting all those years in the waiting room, I also heard women discuss how to deal with the symptoms and side effects of multiple chronic conditions that they had to contend with besides cancer: obesity, diabetes, epilepsy, cardiovascular disease, asthma, gastritis, arthritis, and chronic fatigue syndrome.

After the cancer had metastasized, Laurene became even more resolved to enjoy life in as many positive ways as possible. During the balance of 1999, we enjoyed every day together, and looked for what Laurene called her daily miracles. We both changed how we anticipated small pleasures, experienced life, and expressed ourselves.

For example, we established little healing rituals. We embraced after each time I had to raise her to a standing position from either the car seat or a wheel chair. We wrote in our journals. We talked about how to alter Laurene's lifelong tendency to overwork, and her predisposition to worry. We looked for ways to relax. We walked every day we could, and looked for lucky pennies as we did. In the evenings, we would swim naked in our pool with the fountains going full blast, with Jimmy Buffet's "Cheeseburger in Paradise" blaring through the speakers. At these times, or after a phone call from the girls, Laurene and I felt a radiance like we lived in a world for which we were not created—a disease-free world without work or worries or weariness. I rubbed her feet with peppermint oil every night before bed.

The intimacy of our married life up to this point had been limited by the demands of two jobs and four children. Now cancer had thrown us back on ourselves to the special times we had spent while dating, and on our honeymoon. It would be difficult to say that we were spending a second honeymoon during Laurene's treatments, but in a way it was true. We were together now all the time. Like her doctor, I knew where I could touch her body without causing her pain. I examined her wounds to see how they were healing. I knew her body more thoroughly than when I had looked upon it as a container for her energy, a structure for her clothes, or a playground for sex.

I don't know exactly when it happened, but at some point, caring for Laurene changed from a task to a joy.

I noticed the subtle changes in her face and limbs, the changing texture of her hair, the new way she balanced her body with the weight of one breast rather than two, the slight droop of her left eyelid from what we later learned to be an optic tumor metastasis. I observed how the shape of Laurene's nose matched the shape of her mother's nose, and how her patterns of speech and expressions mirrored her father's way of talking. Most of all, I learned to read the unspoken language of her face: the face of pain, the face of anger, the face of fear, the face of anticipation, the face of resignation, the face of prayer. And when she did speak, I felt privileged to hear the words that had resided concealed in her heart, as if I was the first and only person to hear them in the history of the world.

We couldn't make the cancer go away, but we could manage how we lived with cancer. We both believed in this strategy, and it worked for a long time. Even though five different chemotherapies and over one hundred total hours of radiation ransacked her body, Laurene never had a serious infection during her cancer treatment. She had had no communicable diseases—no flu, no colds in eleven years. Her doctors had predicted that she would most likely die of a catastrophic occurrence like a heart attack, hemorrhage, or infection. None of that happened. Laurene had a concise explanation for her resilience. "I have been loved. There are so many people in the world who suffer and haven't been loved like me."

Beginning in 2000, Laurene's overall stamina and resilience began to drop. Her physical balance was off, in part from losing her left breast. She fell once in a while, and in one case, hit her head on a marble floor in our home and bled profusely. When I met her at the Emergency Room, she told me she had always been clumsy, and laughed it off. Weariness also set in. She would say over and over again when resting, *"I've got to get up. I've got to get up."* Everything took more effort.

As we both tired from eight years of Laurene's treatment, we felt less confident about our ability to deal with events. The out-of-pocket medical expenses began to exceed $10,000 a year. I sold what we could do without, liquidated my 401k, and took a lump sum early withdrawal on my pension. Just deciphering the long pages of itemized charges took days, and meetings with the accounting staff at the clinic. When Laurene was occupied receiving therapy or routine treatments, I used the time to get away when I felt overloaded. Filling prescriptions, juggling up to four days of clinic appointments a week, taking care of the house, sitting endless hours in waiting rooms, keeping people informed of what was going on with Laurene —everything piled up.

I knew that I loved Laurene just as much as always, but I was tired and mad and frustrated with the cancer. I felt like a scuffed up old shoe. I wanted my old life back. I missed the respect, power, and influence of an executive position along with feelings of pride and accomplishment at the end of a work day. I even missed the bad stuff about business: the politics, the flattery, the false optimism, the illusion of control, and other unattractive features of corporate life. And I was vaguely upset with myself. Was I hiding something behind Laurene's disease? Was I shirking the hard work of making a living? Was I incompetent as a provider, husband, caregiver, father? Was I in some way a fraud, hiding behind the persona of a self-sacrificing spouse?

The year 2000 was a low point for both of us. The doctors always had something new to try, but we began to think they were merely casting about with experimental drugs, and each new regimen had its own set of unknown risks and consequences, and a new set of side effects. Ending a particular chemotherapy would be a temporary relief, before the next one began. The time at the clinic increased from once a month to once a week to three or more days per week. We visited new clinics and departments to see dentists, dermatologists, ophthalmologists, neurologists, bone specialists, physical therapists, and pain management specialists.

After we bottomed out by thinking that we were helpless, things began to improve. Not only did Laurene's blood markers show signs of remission, but our attitudes turned around. We finally realized that we couldn't maneuver our way out alone in what seemed like a hostile universe of uncontrollably growing cancer cells. When we gave up trying to control the outcome of the disease, we began to appreciate what was around us—the clinic staff, our friends, our family, and each other. We asked for and received help, rather than relying on our own resources, our own will power, and our own actions.

More than anything, Laurene and I stopped managing our lives, and began living our lives!

For years, people told us "we're praying for you," but I failed to take their offers seriously. I heard their intentions more like "have a nice day," or "good luck to you." For the first time, I thought that perhaps the prayers were working, and that even though we didn't feel saved or redeemed, even though we were not becoming better persons from the struggle, God was somewhere on the other side of our suffering, nudging us forward and keeping us safe.

LESSON EIGHT

Suffering is not God's way of perfecting us.

9.

*"Surely we're meant to win this battle," he
    began,
"Unless...But we were offered help...
Look how long it's taking for someone to come!"*

Dante's Inferno, Canto IX

One afternoon on our way back home from a treatment, I had to pull onto feeder roads off Route 45 twice for Laurene to vomit. A dead mutt sprawled across the bloody concrete with its guts spilling out. After I cleaned Laurene up, she said, "Everyone's going to die. I just have more information about when." Leave it to Laurene to see looming death as a data point. But she was right. She had completed nine experimental chemotherapies, and the cancer still advanced. Her blood counts could no longer endure more chemotherapy, even if another one had been an option.

As we experienced a downward trend in Laurene's prospects for long-term survival, we felt a loss of control over the disease. But her everyone's-going-to-die statement was the first time she had admitted death to her vocabulary. Ironically, the Gallery Furniture billboard *(**GALLERY FURNITURE SAVES YOU MONEY!**)* stood like a big movie screen across from where we were parked.

"I can't get up from the chair in the family room anymore," Laurene said. "I need to buy one of those electric lift chairs from that guy. I bet they cost an arm and a leg." The next week, we bought a chair. The floor salesman made the mistake of telling Laurene that the price was not negotiable. We ended up buying the chair for a nice discount, but we had to go see Mattress Mack first, the guy on the North Freeway billboard holding a fist of money that he promised to save customers. Laurene wanted her fistful.

Beyond the assistance of a lift recliner, we realized that we now needed to reengineer our entire survival strategy. End of life care had to be part of the new strategy, and after Laurene considerations formed in both our minds. We also needed to start drawing the wagons around our daughters. We had not shared all the details of what was happening, because we wanted them to go about their lives with little or no interruptions to their education or careers. We had also limited what we had asked of others. I called Bob, my hunting buddy in Houston, and told him that I need to talk with him more often. He began to call me or have lunch with me every week. I joined the Anderson Network to connect with other men whose wives had a similar diagnosis to Laurene's.

We had deferred examining our faith in any greater depth than what might come to mind during a weekly church service. We started receiving pastoral counseling from an assistant minister at our church.

What else helped turn us around after we had bottomed out?

Deep Caring

Beyond her immediate friends and family, Laurene strengthened connections to all the people around her. These relationships kept her from feeling isolated, and gave her a daily source of positive support. Some distant acquaintances wrote letters, or traveled to Houston for visits. People prayed for her. One woman volunteered to research clinical trials. One served as our travel agent when we could get away for trips. People brought food to the house—soup, lots of soup. Another woman would drive Laurene to appointments, shop with her, and help her plan special events like birthday and graduation parties for our children. Sharon, a lifelong buddy from grade school, helped Laurene wrap birthday and Christmas gifts. Sharon frequently invited Laurene to her home on a nearby lake for a day of relaxation. Laurene appreciated these rest and recovery days, because she felt pampered and appreciated. I would often come along and also benefit from the loving attention of a good friend.

I want to mention another special woman, another close friend of Laurene's. Ellen lived in College Station, Texas, a one-and-half hour drive from our house. Every Thursday morning for three years, Ellen would get up early, and pull in our driveway around eight thirty in the morning. I could do anything I wanted until five. Sometimes I would golf with a friend or go fishing on Lake Conroe. Once in a while, I would bike to a park, and sit on a park bench. Or simply do errands like shopping for groceries. This weekly respite helped immensely. It helped me reclaim a part of my life before the cancer. I had been a caregiver for going on ten years. I needed some breaks.

In addition to recreation, I needed to deal with my ambivalent feelings. There was an emotional war raging in my head: guilt (she has cancer, not me), sadness (we'll never retire together), anger (I've lost my career) (I hate cancer), loneliness (people pay more attention to her than to me), jealousy (healthy couples don't know how good they have it), and annoyance (I'm tired of cleaning up messes). I felt trapped in a struggle that appeared to be unending. I was getting plain tired, sometimes bored, sometimes overwhelmed. When I returned home each week, I would walk Ellen out to her car and thank her. She would say it's nothing at all. It was more than she knew.

Ellen, who more than anyone was my personal caregiver, died of breast cancer a few years ago. I miss her. Even though we didn't spend much time together, I appreciated her loving support for both Laurene and me. Her entire adult life, she had wanted a cabin in Maine, her home state. She finally purchased a place shortly before her diagnosis. Her battle was short compared to ours.

Why do we keep losing so many good women to breast cancer? Why? Why? Why? Someday I want one of my granddaughters to say to her daughter, "Your great grandpa wrote a book about when women used to die from breast cancer."

The Healing Web

In addition to near and dear friends, Laurene assembled a large group of supporters in a circle of support outside the innermost circle of her family and close friends. I counted them—150 plus. She scheduled weekly therapeutic massage appointments, and when she could no longer manage to travel to the studio, the therapist came to our house with a portable massage table. Reflexologists, counselors, physical therapists, and yoga instructors supported her over the years of her cancer treatment. These people played many different roles: experts, advice-givers, cheerleaders, confidants, spiritual guides, and prayer warriors.

As Laurene became increasingly disabled, we used a combination of walkers and wheelchairs to convey her from one place to another, both inside and outside the house. I learned how to maneuver the wheelchair with skill, and to assemble and disassembled it quickly. Each week, I wheeled

Laurene into a classroom in our church for women's bible study. I noticed a number of women sitting beside huge spiral-bound notebooks with colorful tabs along with thick study bibles. The leader opened with a long prayer spoken from the heart, and followed with a selection of soulful contemporary music. The only man in a women's bible study didn't appear to bother anyone, so I began to prepare for the meetings and participate. Laurene wasn't the only woman in the group going through life challenges. The women talked about illnesses and addictions, problems with work and family, and their spiritual questions. During these meetings, we developed a perspective of how everyone has tough life challenges of one kind or another. These kind women cheered us up every week.

Also, on the first Sunday of each month, we attended an evening healing service at our church. I felt calmer and lighter after the services, like the burden of what we were going through was more bearable. Somehow it was important for us to feel, speak, and be seen when we were most vulnerable. I felt like we weren't struggling alone. I also felt more connected to Laurene as the joyful person I loved behind her pain and separate from her suffering, the person I loved with cancer in the background, and with our relationship unaffected by the disease. As we held hands in the sanctuary, Laurene said we're just two turkeys who love each other.

The Healing Village

In addition to individual relationships, we gained support through other groups, some of which had nothing to do with cancer. For example, we registered for "Introduction to Spanish" at the local community college. Our professor loved to teach, and we enjoyed the mental challenge and interactions with the other students. Helping one of the young Spanish students with his homework gave Laurene satisfaction. She felt useful and enjoyed engaging with people, both those who were facing similar health challenges, and those whose lives were not involved in dealing with illnesses of any kind.

Laurene attended the *Rosebuds* breast cancer support group, and later, *Rosebuds II* for breast cancer survivors with metastatic cancer. She returned from these meetings with a renewed will to survive, and with lots of practical advice on everything from treatment side effects to new treatment protocols and clinical trials. The group celebrated all types of milestones—birthdays, anniversaries, and years of survival.

These communal experiences gave us a sense of connection to others, and helped us understand that we were not alone in what we were experiencing. In addition to a sense of belonging, these activities gave Laurene and me opportunities to provide support to others. When you receive so much help, it's helpful to find small ways to give back.

Brief Encounters

Beyond her family, friends, and acquaintances, Laurene looked for other opportunities to connect with people every day. At the clinic, she counseled other women who were dealing with breast cancer, people she just happened to run into in the cafeteria or the waiting rooms. She never turned down an opportunity to chat with strangers whom she would meet in stores and shops. She loved children, and would smile and talk with them as well as adults. This kind of support had value for both her and others. For Laurene, it was a way to expand and extend her life, and to add meaning, purpose, and beauty to each day.

The benefit of brief encounters also happened during our travels. During our earlier trip to Asia, as we had tried to carry our luggage up and down steep stairs to get from Narita Airport to the bullet train bound for Kyoto, a Japanese businessman observed Laurene trying to drag her roller bag up the steps. He bowed, and then took over. He guided us to the train. Laurene not only thanked him, but asked what he did for a living. He sold electronic organs for Yamaha. He was a father with four children. His help enlivened Laurene. She talked about him all the way to Kyoto. He was a healer as well as a businessman.

A Husband's Passage Through Cancerland

Once on the train, I benefited from another brief encounter. I was starved, and purchased two bento lunch boxes before we boarded the train. Once in my seat, I opened the beautifully packaged lunch, and started to eat the decorative green rice paper I thought was some form of Japanese lettuce. A teenage girl sitting with another girl her age in a seat across from us, stood up and approached me. She smiled and bowed politely over my tray of food. She picked up a piece of the rice paper, and turned her head sideways. We later helped the girls with their English homework. Kindness heals.

Near the end of the trip that included Tokyo, Beijing, and Hong Kong, Laurene was exhausted. We were dragging our roller bags to a gate, and I noticed that her shoelace was untied. I didn't want her to fall. "Laurene, stop, we need to tie your shoelaces."

"I'll wait until I fall down," she said. "Then I won't have to bend over so far."

She never allowed me to do anything that she could do for herself, but I ignored her and tied her shoelaces in a double knot (she hated double knots).

LESSON NINE

Help comes in many forms and in unexpected ways.

10.

*'I only keep my deepest thoughts to myself,' I
   said,
'In order not to talk too much,
As you yourself have warned me more than once.'*

Dante's Inferno, Canto X

Healing in the Waiting Room

One day, I had been sitting in a clinic waiting room for six hours. I had tired of reading. I had run to the clinic pharmacy and back twice to fill prescriptions. I had eaten breakfast and lunch in the cafeteria. I had updated my to-do list. I couldn't think of a single other thing to do. So I looked around me, and listened to the buzz of conversation. "Where are you from?" "How did you find out?" "What's your schedule for today?" "Did you have to fill out this form?" "Who wants to have sex when you hurt all over?" "I can't get anti-depressants, but dark chocolate works," "Did you know you can choose your own color for a new nipple?" "They told me they got it all, but they didn't." "What did you tell your daughter about genetics?" "I just graduated to annual check-ups."

I observed patients giving gifts to other patients—inspirational books, hand-made bookmarks, and healthy snacks. I watched as doctors emerged from their offices to check the news on the TV. A few times, I overheard doctors conducting an appointment in the waiting room. I didn't know if the patient had no health insurance, or if there had been an appointment scheduling problem, but the doctor was discussing treatment, writing prescriptions, and counseling the woman—he was practicing medicine in the waiting room. Nurses, social workers, and volunteers walked around chatting and laughing. People helped each other, and exchanged information on everything from recipes to clinical trials. They told their stories to each other. Rather than a place to sit and fight off boredom, I started to see the waiting room with new eyes.

I felt like I was watching the daily activities of a small, crowded village. People who needed to talk found someone to talk with. I began to regard the place as more than a high traffic public place like an airport lounge or restaurant waiting area. A sacredness drifted into my consciousness. Love and kindness hovered in the air. With this new awareness, my attitude transcended from thinking that healing only took place on the other side of the waiting room walls to the thought that healing also happened in the waiting rooms.

In addition to the patients, perhaps this neutral space was also a place of respite for the doctors and nurses as well. I thought of the possibility that the fifty waiting rooms at MD Anderson could all be filled with healing relationships. Buried in my books and magazines, I had missed the importance of who was around me. From that day forward, I took time to listen and talk to the people sitting around me. I was never disappointed.

Unexpected things happened all the time. One day, a nurse waited for a translator to inform a man and his wife from Argentina about his test results. He had traveled to MD Anderson, because his home doctor had informed him that incurable cancer had overtaken his body, and he would most likely die in a few months. The translator could not be found. The nurse looked like she might burst. Finally, she couldn't wait any longer. She practically shouted in English for all to hear, ***"YOU DON'T HAVE CANCER. YOU HAVE ARTHRITIS!"*** A Latina woman was sitting nearby, and translated for the couple. All the people in the waiting room stood up and cheered. People wanted a future with hope. Hopeful events happened all the time—what Laurene called daily miracles.

Unlike my experience in typical doctor's offices, current magazines replaced out-of-date ones, and the magazines reflected a wide range of interests rather than a particular doctor's personal hobbies. The snack cart rumbled by every half hour or so. Games and puzzles and books were available. The rooms were well-lighted, the walls were painted with soft colors, and the chairs and sofas were comfortable. People talked and slept. Conversations ranged from how to get around the clinic to alternative healing practices. People sat on the chairs or cross-legged on the floor. And if you had time and wanted to get away from others, a Patient and Family Room provided a place where you could go to rest. A volunteer would greet you at the door with a pillow and blanket, and guide you to a dark room filled with assorted recliners and sofas. The volunteers covered you with the blanket, then asked when you wanted to be leave. Silence ruled.

People rolled by on stretchers, in wheelchairs, with walkers, or speed-walking in jogging suits. Over the decade that I spent in these waiting rooms, I developed a sense of how everyday life blended with the divine, a deeper awareness of what I had earlier experienced while sipping tea in Kyoto. Once while walking by rooms in the hospital wing, I observed a man with long, wild white hair sitting upright on his hospital bed with a tranquil look on his face. A pale-yellow light flooded his room. The sight stopped me in my tracks. There was no way I could have prefabricated this awareness. I wasn't expecting to see a man with the godlikeness of Einstein sitting in a golden glowing room. For the rest of the day, I felt unusually calm and alert. I carried the golden light and the image of the man in and around me like a portable aura. Maybe that's what it means to behold something?

"Behold, I bring you great tidings...from an old man sitting in his bed."

The Healing Team

On the other side of the doors leading from the waiting rooms, were rabbit warrens of tiny patient examination rooms. Here the healing teams resided. Laurene had appointed herself CEO of her healing team. There was no question who was in charge. Her personal management of professional support relationships served her as another important dimension of her survivorship. The doctors called Laurene their light, because of her resilience in dealing with cancer. One day I found a clinic note in Laurene's medical file that read: "Mrs. Evans is well known in our department for management of metastatic breast cancer."

Laurene also developed good working relationships with other medical professionals in the various departments of the clinic from pain management to physical therapy. She stressed the importance of nurses. "Be tough on the doctors, but easy on the nurses," she said. Nurses could help her in ways doctors could not—from showing female nurses the location of sores too embarrassing to show the male doctors, to asking for medical advice that she had forgotten to mention during a scheduled appointment. The nurses also helped navigate the scheduling bureaucracy. Nurses helped Laurene clarify how to describe her symptoms and collect her thoughts, so that the doctor meetings could be more efficient and useful. They were also the first to respond to emergencies, and orchestrate life-saving responses. During these years, I would sometimes need to call *"NURSE!"* A nurse was always there, running to our assistance.

Much of the support had nothing to do with Laurene. It was available to everyone. One day we needed to rush from one part of the clinic to the other for a test that had to be done before a surgery scheduled for the next morning. It was about seven in the evening. I had already chased down Laurene's three-foot-high medical file that commanded its own seat in a wheelchair like a crotchety patient spitting paper clips on the floor. I rushed the medical file to the correct department, and then returned for Laurene, a lengthy walk down corridors, over sky bridges, up and down elevators.

I rushed along, hoping not to get lost. No place was easy to find in the vast clinic. (Here is an example of one of my typical paths from the main building to the radiation treatment center: From The Aquarium follow signs to Elevator B, take Elevator B to the second floor, follow the signs to Elevator G, take Elevator G back to first floor, follow signs in lobby to Radiation Treatment Center.) Laurene was hooked up to an IV tree, so I had to push her wheel chair down the long hallways with one hand, and keep the IV stand wheeling alongside. To my dismay, the IV lines wrapped around the wheels. They threatened to rip the catheters out. We both panicked. A young doctor who was walking in the opposite direction stopped, calmed us down, and carefully freed the lines. He sent us on our way. We arrived on time for the test, and kept our schedule for surgery the next day.

So Laurene's healing team helped her work the magic of staying well for a long time. There is no question in my mind about the connection between the healing nature of relationships and the immune system's ability to resist the progression of disease. These relationships are universally available and reciprocal. Carl Rogers (1980) describes healing relationships in *A Way of Being* better than I could imagine: "I find that when I am closest to my intuitive, inner self, when I am somehow in touch with the unknown in me, when I am perhaps in a slightly altered state of consciousness, then whatever I do seems to be full of healing."

In addition to the team at MD Anderson, through the research of Kay, one of Laurene's friends from graduate business school, we found a grouchy little man who was doing experimental work with vaccinations to trigger the immune system, the first line of the body's defense against most diseases and unnatural invaders, to destroy cancer cells. Dr. George Springer took on 19 women with terminal breast cancer diagnoses. His office/lab was located at 3333

Out of the Inferno

Green Bay Road in North Chicago. Everyone had to show up on the same day for the vaccines. If you didn't show up, you were thrown out of the program. Women flew into Chicago from across the country. After the vaccinations, patients had to return to the lab in a few weeks to record the results. The doctor had less than admirable interpersonal skills. Foremost, he was a scientist. He was looking for the cure for breast cancer—his T/Tn vaccine therapy. Fortunately, Herta, his assistant, softened our visits with her consideration and warmth.

We began visiting Dr. Springer in 1992. Because the regimen was experimental, we had to pay all expenses. Laurene showed positive reactions to the vaccinations for the next ten years. The FDA shut down Dr. Springer's lab in the mid 1990s. I can't recall the reason, something administrative, but the lab reopened within six months. When Dr. Springer died in 1998, Herta continued giving Laurene the vaccinations. After Laurene was technically disqualified from the study because of her recurrence in 2000, Herta kept giving her the shots. Laurene's last treatment occurred in early July, 2002. The day before our last scheduled visit, Laurene insisted that we drag chairs out to the narrow balcony of a motel lining a busy highway. We watched a grand display of fireworks. "This may be my last Fourth of July," she said. She wasn't melodramatic. She was simply stating a thought.

Of the 19 women in the Phase I Study, all survived five years from diagnosis, and 11 survived for over ten years (Laurene survived for eleven). We don't know if these treatments helped Laurene beat the odds to live longer than expected, but we do know that these treatments gave us hope beyond the therapies at MD Anderson. We also know that Dr. Springer's early experiments attempting to manipulate the immune system in the 1990s are now in the mainstream of leading cancer research. His early aim to harness the body's own immune system to fight cancer was correct. Now cancer therapeutics (checkpoint inhibitor therapies) have been developed to unlock the immune system to recognize and destroy cells carrying mutations. Some patients with widespread metastatic disease have already been rendered cancer free from these therapies.

The hope for a miracle cure for cancer resides in the minds of every person with cancer. The thousands of mostly unknown cancer warriors searching for a cure also give hope to those who deal with cancer as family, nurses, or physicians. Laurene's doctor at MD Anderson knew that she was receiving the injections. He told us that Dr. Springer's research, while unproven, was based on "sound medical principles." Once again, we discovered that the smartest oncologists were also the humblest. Some doctors might have thought that our attempts at alternative treatments showed a lack of confidence in their expertise, but not Laurene's doctor. He did his best with the knowledge that someone else's best might be better.

Even though "the cure" remains elusive, every week there are new discoveries that bring breast cancer closer to treatment as a chronic disease, rather than the death sentence that it once was. And someday, there will be a cure. In the meantime, having the hope of a cure improves the quality of life of breast cancer survivors and most probably extends their lives.

Why wasn't Laurene content to exclusively follow the treatment plans of one of the finest cancer clinic's in the world? Dr. Springer was part of Laurene's personal anti-cancer strategy that extended beyond MD Anderson to learn about and explore all possibilities for survival, and to communicate to others that she intended to survive. She looked for every way to outwit the cancer, and to dodge its blows. Her loose clothes that popped with color and her bright jewelry had replaced the navy blue suits that she had worn to work at General Electric (she no longer wanted to look anonymous). Her demure, professional demeanor at work had also changed in direct response to her illness. She unveiled her powers to persuade, pester, insist, or beg depending on whatever her personal advocacy required. If she offended people in her efforts to live, so be it. Cancer survivors can't always be polite.

In addition to assertive behavior, Laurene could find casual ways of presenting her cancer to others in order not to scare people away. She used humor effectively with a repertoire of funny stories. She constantly referred to her travel plans. Around the house, she kept adding to what she called her "rat piles" of unfinished business—books, magazines, news clippings, research on clinical trials, a community college course catalog, lists of things to do that had nothing to do with cancer. She made herself and her surroundings a wide-screen cinema to broadcast her will to survive. Her strategy flashed and flickered a consistent stream of messages to everyone around her like a billboard on Texas State Route 45:

DON'T GIVE UP ON ME!

I HAVE NEW ADVENTURES PLANNED!

I HAVE THE WIT AND THE WILL AND THE IMAGINATION NOT TO LET CANCER DEFINE MY LIFE! I'M NOT FINISHED!

LESSON TEN

Healing comes from unexpected people and in the most unlikely places.

11.

"We have to wait awhile to adapt
To the noxious fumes—once we do,
They'll no longer bother us."
That's what my teacher said. I said, "Let's find a way
To make use of the delay, so we won't waste time."

Dante's Inferno, Canto XI

Dante had descended into the fourth circle of hell encasing "all the evils of the universe." The higher circles had been tame compared to what he could now see. His teacher refused his request to turn around, and no one would come to rescue him. He felt abandoned. Perhaps he had given up hope. He rested on the edge of a bank filled with enormous broken boulders, and looked down to the deeper circles of the Inferno. He stopped talking.

I had stopped writing. The first ten chapters of manuscript had covered the easy subjects. Even though Laurene had received a grave diagnosis, we did not believe that cancer would kill her. We still hoped that the battle could be won. Bad news was infrequent, and the move to Houston proved new and exciting. I had written about these years with relative ease. I kept nudging myself to go on, but I couldn't seem to write more.

Since Laurene's death, I had written poetry, short stories, and two novels that had allowed me to approach losing Laurene obliquely. The main characters in the novels were both widowers. Maybe this indirect approach of turning my hurt into fiction was the best I could do. Keeping my thoughts and feelings at a distance had carried me along so far. I could get close to my grief, but not too close. I could write made-up stories about what happened. I could leave out the awful stuff. I could skip over the long, slow uninteresting facts of dealing with cancer. I wouldn't have to remember all the horrid cocktails of Laurene's combination chemotherapies. I could invent stories that might be more appealing to write about and to read.

I also wondered whether or not I should proceed head on with such a personal history. What if I hurt people I love? What if dredged up bad memories that my daughters would have preferred to forget? Alan Shapiro in his essay, "Why Write?" described part of my dilemma: "Even the most affectionate portrait of a loved one, the most intimate praise (never mind depictions of estrangement or disaffection) can and will offend." What would Laurene have said if I had told her that I intended to share her private struggles? And how do you explain to your new wife that you are writing a memoir about your old wife?

A Husband's Passage Through Cancerland

One evening, I discovered three cardboard storage boxes in my furnace room filled with photos that Laurene had neatly dated PICTURE BOX1999, PICTURE BOX 2000, and PICTURE BOX 2001. I counted twelve packages of white envelopes containing a total of 491 pictures in the 1999 box alone. Laurene had taken most of these during our July trip to Europe with Jennifer and Meredith. I don't remember ever going through them, but I'm sure that I must have glanced at them shortly after they had been processed. I wanted to see them again. Maybe looking at pictures would help me remember what life had been like for us during the year before things really got difficult? I wanted to write more than a timeline of the trip. I wanted to recapture the mood, tone, and feeling of what had happened. So fifteen years later, I sat down by a window in my office to look through them. As rain poured down on a July afternoon in northern Michigan, I relived our two weeks in Europe.

The three years happened to be those difficult years that I couldn't seem to write about. As I rifled through the photographs, I felt like Laurene's heart was still beating. The memories came back fresh and new. The pictures told stories—Laurene's stories about how precious her life had been and had yet to be. I felt like the pictures might guide me deeper into the passages of the most difficult years of cancer inferno. The cliché about how one picture is worth a thousand words came to mind, but in this case, the pictures helped me find the words I had lost. The photographs showed still life, but behind each picture, I could see movement, moments of laughter and sadness, and recall bits of conversation.

I also realized that of the thousand stories represented in the picture boxes, I needn't write about every one. I could pick the ones that represented the best and worst of what happened. Some of the stories might be embarrassing, uncomfortable, or stressful to remember, but when I realized that I could select the stories, I could continue—readers needn't know every detail about the ups and downs of our marriage, the disturbances to our children, the career and financial problems, the hallucinations and nightmares, the deformities, the nausea, vomiting, and diarrhea. Whitewashing or sanitizing the memoir with manufactured cheer would be a mistake, but slowly drowning readers in the puddles of breast cancer's physical, mental, and emotional side effects would not be helpful either.

Laurene's reputation for family picture-taking was notorious. We had all been dragged into the Olin Mills franchise store for family photos at least once a year since we had been married over ten years earlier. We froze in stiff poses directed by the photographer against painted backgrounds on the wall or screens of fake fireplaces that dropped mechanically from the ceiling. The pictures kept taking over wall space in the house, edging out fine art that, from Laurene's perspective, could not possibly be more beautiful than photographs of people she loved. Laurene told us the color scheme and what to wear, and gave us all coaching on how to hold our heads and how to smile without looking like fakes or like we were bored, which we were.

For our wedding ceremony, Laurene had purchased pink dresses for my daughters and hers. White lace lined the dresses, and the girls wore pink ribbons in their hair, white gloves, wrist corsages, white socks and shoes. Meredith's dress was splattered with mud, because she and her sisters had chased each other around the rain-drenched grounds before the ceremony, and Meredith had fallen trying to keep up with the "big three." Out of the corner of my eye, I kept seeing them run by like chase scenes from Wes Anderson's *Moonrise Kingdom*. They all hated the frilly dresses, and they hated the picture of them all posed in their dresses, taken at Olin Mills with forced demure smiles the day before the wedding. To make it worse, Laurene had individual pictures taken of each girl, and these were hung from the walls of our home. When Laurene wasn't looking, and especially when their friends visited the house, the pictures disappeared from the walls. I kept finding them stashed under their beds opposite picture hooks protruding from the walls.

As I reviewed the pictures, I noticed something different. Laurene had nearly always taken posed pictures like the Olin Mills photographs. I think this was partly because of her Texas upbringing. Many times she had told me, "You don't surprise people," "You don't embarrass people," "You don't make them look like fools," "When you want to take someone's picture, you ask their permission first." Laurene had always preceded the camera click by saying "*one, two, three-hee*" with three an octave higher as a warning to remove unsightly smirks or suffer a mother's wrath. She believed in common courtesy. That's how Neil and Stella had raised her. When Stella died, Laurene omitted Stella's age from the obituary. "Mom, never told her age," Laurene said.

As I looked through nearly 500 snapshot in the 1999 box, there were relatively few posed photos. Laurene had gone freestyle with her camera. She was breaking her own rules. The candid snapshots were fun, whimsical, and beautiful, and not at all like the expressionless, posed photos with the artificial background screens at Olin Mills. Laurene had always complained to me that she wasn't creative. I told her that everyone has different ways of expressing themselves. I could see her inner critic disappearing from the pictures. In her own prudent way, she was becoming wild and reckless with her picture taking. I looked at one example after another.

Meredith stands with her back to Laurene looking out a window over the red tile rooftops of Lucca. From an opening in an ancient stone tower, Jennifer gazes down on the Rhine River. Another photo shows Mer facing the inside of a cathedral window with her body silhouetted by white light coming in from outside. The outline of her thin body makes her look like an angel. Another one shows Mer sunning herself on a patio by a lake in northern Italy. Her legs are tangled up in a folding chair, and she has a silly grin on her face. Others show the girls sleeping. The photos are close-ups, invasions of a teenager's privacy, as if Laurene wanted to see and remember each detail of their faces.

Still another photo captures the two sisters standing on a river bridge under an ornate lamppost. Laurene's stealthy camera catches each of them singly or together reading books, eating omelets, fondues, and pretzels; shopping for chocolates, napping in the car (including a nap photo of Meredith sleeping with her nose snubbed up against the car window). One photo shows the girls sitting in a dark dining room with their faces lit by a large candle. The last photo from the box shows Jennifer and Meredith perched in the prow of a gondola in Venice. These were not photographs lit by backlighting, but by a mother's love.

Some of Laurene's photographs followed patterns. For example, she loved to take pictures of McDonald's restaurants in every country where we traveled. Laurene had a weakness for fast food; probably because of all the hard-boiled eggs her mother had given her on the weekly car trips from

Houston to Brownwood and back when she was a little girl. She loved to capture the menus in different languages (SUPERPREIS MENU, I NOSTRIE McMENU). She marveled at a McDonald's embedded in train car that passed through a Swiss village twice a day. She couldn't believe that there was a McDonald's at the Matterhorn where a shepherd herded his goats past the entrance, and another one in Florence amid the beautiful cathedrals and museums. She also took pictures of menu boards outside other restaurants. During the whole trip, Laurene was feeling well, so she was hungry for food. She was also hungry for life in all its forms, and she took pictures as if photo ops appeared everywhere she looked.

Laurene studied photography as a new hobby. I thought about my Aunt Alma who had started taking piano lessons a few months before she had died of breast cancer. She lived in Athens, Ohio in a large brick house on College Street when I was a freshman at Ohio University. When I visited her, I sat on the piano bench with her while she played. I thought, *why would you take up piano lessons when you knew you were going to die soon?* Now I understood what I could not understand at age seventeen. Laurene lived lifetimes each day, and each lifetime included new interests and new people. And each day filled with goodness. She didn't want to wait for an eternal glory after endless years of suffering. She wanted her little hells followed by little glories. She was greedy that way.

As if to emphasize her awareness of time passing, Laurene took pictures of clock towers everywhere, from the campanile in the Piazza San Marco in Florence to the robin's egg blue bell towers in small Swiss towns. She also photographed statues of saints, and numerous photos of Michelangelo's David—his full nude front, his overly large right hand, and his round butt, tensed in readiness to battle Goliath. I was jealous. Michelangelo carved David's ass out of a piece of marble. God made my ass. Nevertheless, Laurene liked to call me "turkey butt." Of all her pet names for me, I liked this one the least.

She photographed a gondolier on the Grand Canal in Venice with his billowing white shirt and tight black pants. Standing on the stern of the gondola, his pose is strikingly similar to Michelangelo's David. Laurene also took pictures of mountains, lakes, waterfalls, and rivers. I found one of Zermatt with its snowy peaks fading into the white light of mist and clouds. Another shows the flowered footbridges over the Rhine in Luzern. Still another frames a fountain of green gargoyles spewing water out of their mouths. Each snapshot was like a kiss—a kiss to the earth, a kiss to the sky, a kiss to us. Hello and good-bye kisses.

Laurene liked the complex and exuberant colors of Marc Chagall, her favorite artist. She treasured a plate book of his paintings, illustrations, drawings, and lithographs. A framed print of Chagall's

Cornflowers hung in our house filled with yellows and radiant cornflower blues. Her photographs displayed colors bursting with life—a red and white hot air balloon sailing over fields of grain through patches of white clouds and deep blue sky, the inside of a chocolate shop with red, yellow, blue, and orange wrapping, and gardens of flowers—varieties of roses, hydrangeas, hibiscus, and dahlias. Sadly, there were also photos of flowers in graveyards, most often pictures of the recent gravestones. Was she shopping for one?

And in her perpetual loyalty to the entire family, at the end of the last package of envelopes, Laurene included a snapshot of our larger-than-life cat, Brother Butterscotch. She took the picture after she returned to Houston, out of fairness to another member of our family who had not been to Europe, but could not be left out. She had not asked Bro's permission. He was sleeping on his side, although I'm not exactly sure if he had what you would call a side. He certainly was not in a posed position.

Our trip to Europe in 1999 was not simply a trip to celebrate Meredith's high school graduation. It was the beginning of Laurene's long goodbye. Her way of saying goodbye made heaven part of ordinary life, and set ordinary life free. She took liberties like Chagall when he had painted a pale blue girl flying over the Eiffel Tower embracing a lamb.

One evening as we sat in Portofino watching the boats dock, Laurene surprised us by ordering an expensive bottle of Prosecco in a silver bucket of ice. She told us to sip slowly to make it last.

After sifting through the picture boxes, I once again appreciated what had made life worth living for Laurene. Reliving those joyful moments enlivened my will to resume writing. But my new writing had a different purpose. My old purpose had been falsely therapeutic, a way to get over a life that had ceased. My new purpose was to preserve a story for its own sake: to tell my wife's story, to describe my own part in her story, and to make what I had to say the common story of how we seek to discover strength and joy during difficult times.

Out of the Inferno

LESSON ELEVEN

Never let go of what gives you joy.

12.

*The embankment we had to climb down was
  steep.
Like Mont Blanc, but—even worse—what was
  there
Would make anyone want to hide his or her eyes.*

Dante's Inferno, Canto XII

After we returned from Europe, Laurene began a new treatment regimen that resulted in extreme pain but no improvement. The weekly Taxol chemotherapy debilitated her. I realized that she would soon need full-time care. I requested a leave of absence from Intuit, and also informed them that I might not return. Intuit granted me a family medical leave from November 1999 through February 2000. At the end of the leave, I confirmed that I would have to resign. Intuit continued my pay and benefits for six months as part of an on-call consulting agreement. I will always be grateful for their generosity. The company had a big heart. I still have Intuit logo wear emblazoned with the slogan, ***IT'S THE PEOPLE!***

The holding on and letting go process that Laurene had begun in Europe continued into 2000. We both began a grieving process. Although Laurene had always regarded herself as a survivor, one of the people on the tail end of the curve who beats the odds, we experienced a gentle inevitability about the future, like the first snowflakes that fall in advance of a heavy winter storm. In *Blue Nights,* Joan Dideon (2011) wrote: "This book is called 'Blue Nights' because at the time I began it I found my mind turning increasingly to illness, to the end of promise, the dwindling of the days, the inevitability of the fading, the dying of the brightness, but they are also its warning."

By the summer of 2000, I had received my last pay stub from Intuit, and even with excellent health coverage for another few months through COBRA, the unreimbursed medical costs were beginning to rise. We had sold the condo in Los Gatos, but the loss of income concerned me. About this time, I started attending technology forums at Rice University in Houston. The rise of internet companies was reaching a peak. Many of my friends had already invested in dot.com startups, ignoring the warnings of irrational exuberance during the Internet bubble. I talked with Laurene about making some investments for what I thought would be quick returns.

Neil had asked Stella similar questions in the 1950s when he wanted to buy some commercial property in Houston. That property would later turn out to be worth millions, but Stella had resisted. She had lived through the Great Depression, and had insisted that Neil pay off the small mortgage on their house instead. Stella had witnessed too many crying children sitting on their front porches with furniture stacked in the yard. She always thought that the next Depression was right around the corner. She didn't want to lose her house to a banker. Laurene gave me a more nuanced response than her mother's. She told me I could invest as much money as I wanted in start-ups after I paid off the mortgage on our house. I listened to my wife. For the first time in my life, I owned a mortgage-free house.

Even with the mortgage paid off, Meredith's tuition, room, and board at Vanderbilt added up to astronomical bills. I had worked my way through college by stocking shelves in a grocery store, working as a movie theater usher, and serving as a resident assistant in a dormitory. Things had changed. Summer jobs could no longer pay for a college education. I decided to set up a consulting business. I found three companies in Austin and Houston that would pay me a monthly retainer to provide human resources and strategic business planning support. I worked with my laptop sitting beside Laurene in the infusion therapy rooms. Laurene was happy that I had something worthwhile to do besides taking care of her. I enjoyed working again in the familiar territory of my business career.

The bony metastases did not go away. The CT scans showed the cancer eating away at the bones, but we kept getting good news—the blood tests, although primitive by today's standards, showed no evidence of tumor markers in the bloodstream. A year after our European vacation, Laurene began a clinical trial, a Zoledronate vs. Aredia Study. For a time, it appeared that the new chemotherapy might work, but it only worked for a few months. The clinical trial was followed by three additional chemotherapies: Xeloda, Doxil, and cyclophosphamide. By this time, her medical record nearly exceeded what would fit in a wheel chair. It kept getting lost between appointments. I doggedly tracked the records down, and then wheeled the pile, like an overweight patient, to the next waiting room on Laurene's schedule.

During this time, we visited the clinic for appointments an average of four days per week. Often, I would have to pull off Route 45 for Laurene to vomit by the side of the road. She vomited in stores and restaurants, as well as at home and at the clinic, our second home. I carried plastic grocery bags in my pocket all the time. I even got used to the smell of vomit, and rarely gagged. Laurene lost her hair for a third time. The new hair was curly and white. Laurene started wearing more colorful clothes and scarves. She had assembled a wardrobe from Shepherds of Australia filled with her favorite Chagall colors: blues, reds, oranges, greens, yellows, and pinks. Her outfits comprised blouses, slacks, and long dresses with beautifully whimsical designs with stripes, curves, flowers and animals. Most of the outfits displayed three or more colors, a far cry from the dark suits that she had called her corporate uniforms.

Looking through Laurene's 2000 PICTURE BOX, I was amazed at what we managed to do during the year. In January, Intuit gave us a going away party in California, and during the trip, we drove up and down Napa, stopping for a picnic lunch on the Silverado Trail, and later dining at The French Laundry Restaurant. The next day, we followed the 17-mile drive from Pacific Grove to Pebble Beach, taking in the ocean views presented by the Monterrey Peninsula. Another day, we visited Sausalito and Tiburon. For us, California provided an escape to beauty and love without our struggles in Texas. Even the air we breathed was cooler, cleaner, lighter, and dryer than the humid Gulf Coast.

In February, we celebrated Laurene's fifty-third birthday, our thirteenth wedding anniversary in September, my birthday in November, and all of the girls' birthdays through the rest of the year. We visited Meredith at Vanderbilt, and held parties for her high school friends during the school breaks. We visited Laura who had moved to Colorado Springs. By now, both Jennifer and Laura had serious boyfriends, so there were many pictures of the handsome boys that they would soon marry.

Laurene wanted to have fun on every birthday and every holiday. She loved to decorate the house, and hang funny signs from the walls. She had a drawer in the laundry room dedicated to birthday candles, both old and new. There was a large "4" from one of the children's long past birthdays. Throwing a candle away, in her mind, would be like throwing away a memory. I chuckled when I saw a picture of John blowing out his birthday candles. How many women invite their ex-husbands to a party on their birthday? John and I had become friends. He was part of our blended family. I think that Laurene included John partly for Jennifer and Meredith's sake. It made life easier for them to have their father around rather than shuttling back and forth between separate worlds. She didn't want them to grow up in a "broken home." John began to help us with Meredith's college expenses.

When the two of us were alone on Easter, Laurene hid candy-filled plastic Easter eggs in the backyard, and then sent me out to hunt for them. They were filled with my favorite licorice jelly beans, and miniature Snickers Bars. She followed me around the yard, laughing and providing me with clues. She kept count until I found the last egg under the magnolia tree. I felt a rush of childhood excitement, and gave her a long, gentle hug. For a moment, I experienced what my daughters must have felt of Laurene's mothering love for them. I opened one of the eggs, and popped a licorice jellybean in my mouth, then gave her a licorice kiss. Rituals were important to her, and if the children were absent, she still wanted her rituals. Of course, she took pictures.

A Husband's Passage Through Cancerland

We received visits from out-of-town friends (Massachusetts, Ohio, Seattle), and Laurene's Texas friends from high school and college. We took the out-of-town visitors to Brennan's Restaurant for brunch, to the Houston Rodeo, to the Hill Country around Austin, and down to the beach at Galveston for lunches of lump crabmeat, pecan-crusted catfish, and Gulf oysters at Gaido's Seafood Restaurant.

In June, Dave and Marty, my younger brother and sister-in-law, organized a family reunion in Atlanta. We flew to Atlanta with our four daughters, and joined my brother's family. Mom and Dad drove up from Florida. Laurene could still walk for short distances, but she was losing strength. She made it part way up Stone Mountain, then sat down to rest under her white straw hat, while the rest of us climbed to the top. She didn't want to miss a thing. We visited the Coca Cola Museum, the State Capitol, and Underground Atlanta. Even though she was tired, Laurene had also scheduled a visit to the Vanderbilt Estate in Asheville, one more spot on the long bucket list she had created since her cancer diagnosis.

Laurene's priorities had shifted from 1999 to 2000. Rather than seeing the world, she wanted to surround herself with family and friends. I did notice something else. The photographs in Laurene's 2000 picture box were no longer marked with her meticulous pencil codes, and the photos began to be mixed with 1999 and 2001 pictures laying in the 2000 box. Her index cards with columns for date, subject/occasion, place, and comments were blank. There were fewer reorders with cropping instructions. There were also many reprints remaining in the box, as if she had intended to send out duplicates but hadn't had time to put them in the mail. There were also fewer candid shots, and fewer negative adjustments. But Laurene still took pictures of Jennifer and Meredith sleeping. She could never pass one of them sleeping without wanting to record their slumbers forever. Sleeping children are always beautiful, especially to their parents, even when they drool.

I also found two snapshots of the rental car we used in Atlanta. Laurene had discovered that the front fender was about to fall off, and she wanted documentation if we had a problem with the rental agency. Perhaps she was exercising her girlhood fantasy to become a lawyer. She loved to be an advocate for herself or her family. When we were dating, she had contested a traffic ticket in court. The ticket had been issued to her for rolling through a stop sign. She presented photographs of the intersection showing that it was impossible to see cross traffic from the white pavement markers. When she lost, she was miffed. Another time, I had cut the sleeve of my shirt on a sharp object in a Fredericksburg, Texas antique shop. I casually showed her my shirt after I had left the shop. She took me by the hand, and dragged me back into the shop like I was a little boy.

She demanded that the store owner buy me a new shirt. The owner looked at her in disbelief. We didn't get a new shirt, but the owner agreed to move the sharp object off the aisle.

When one of Laurene's critters was hurt, she turned fierce and unrelenting in our defense. She wanted to protect us from every possible harm.

Out of the Inferno

LESSON TWELVE

The photographs you take are like letters written to yourself.

13.

No green leaves, only mono-gray;
No straight limb, only gnarled and tangled;
No fruit, only thorn with poison tips.

Dante's Inferno, Canto XIII

In October 2000, Laurene's left arm broke from a pathological fracture. Blood work and CT Scans showed that the current cocktail of chemotherapies (cyclophosphamide, Doxil, and Xeloda) no longer worked. There seemed to be endless untested new chemotherapies to try if the current ones failed, but each new drug brought on a new set of side effects and secondary consequences. Laurene's doctor recommended infusions of Paclitaxel, a chemotherapy developed from the bark of the Pacific yew. Hardly a targeted therapy, Paclitaxel was also used to treat ovarian, lung, and pancreatic cancers. In November, a one-month treatment break gave us a chance to exercise Laurene's wanderlust for travel one more time. Against the advice of her doctor, she wanted a trip to the English countryside.

We rented a car in London, and followed a map to Gloucestershire through leaden fall skies heavy with rain. Our plan was to follow a route leading to Cornwall, and then back to London. Near the beginning of the trip, we stayed overnight in

Cheltenham, and the next day, drove through The Cotswolds to a little village called Birdlip (I love that name). We arrived in what William Morris had once described as the most beautiful village in the Cotswolds.

Each small cottage with flower boxes below the windows looked like a warm place that you could enter and stay forever. We had intended to look around for a place to lunch before driving on to Cirencester. I left Laurene in the car while I walked into a gift shop to ask for dining suggestions. As I crossed the street, I noticed how everything around me appeared off square—the rooflines of the cottages, the tilted doors and window frames, and the crooked stone walls that followed a crooked river.

After a brief chat with a shopkeeper, I returned to an empty car. It had started to rain, and the wind seemed to be coming from all directions. On the other side of a black stone wall, I heard Laurene screaming for help. I couldn't see her until I had climbed over the wall that separated the car park from the main street of the village. Laurene lay sprawled on her side holding her right arm. When I reached her, I could see that she had scraped her face. She was bleeding. Her blouse and slacks were covered with blood and dirt. She had lost a shoe. Her arm bent at an odd angle. She began to cry. We were both soaked from the rain.

A Husband's Passage Through Cancerland

Laurene had left the car with her camera in hand, and climbed the stone wall to take a picture. The street side of the wall stood twice as high as the wall facing the car park. She had managed to climb to the top of the wall, but lost her balance. She had toppled into the street. As I bent down to help her, I heard a car engine whirring from the direction of a blind curve. I had no time to be gentle. I grabbed her under her arm pits and dragged her to the curb as the driver of a Jaguar hit the brakes, and then zoomed out of sight. It had been so close that I could see the car's steel mesh grillwork. Laurene babbled something about being clumsy. Her face looked white. I thought she might be in shock.

We sat on the curb for a few minutes to get our bearings. The doors and windows of the cottages opened, and people emerged to offer help. We happened to be sitting outside a pub. I carefully raised Laurene to her feet, and we walked inside where an innkeeper brought us cold water and a bag of ice for Laurene's arm. There was no question that her arm was broken. The pub owner provided directions to the nearest hospital in Burford. He gave us bread and cheese, but would take no money. I brought the car around to the pub entrance, and managed to get Laurene strapped in and as comfortable as possible.

During the sixteen-mile drive, Laurene didn't have much to say other than ***RATS!*** She looked cold, so I covered her with my coat. I was still concerned about shock. Even though I worried about her, I felt grateful that we hadn't been run over by the Jaguar. I also felt a vague sense of pride after all the years of feeling helpless about the unstoppable forces of the cancer. *Here was something I could do. I had swooped her up in my arms from the street. I had carried her to safety. I was now driving her to the hospital. I would take care of her for the rest of the trip. At least for moment, I was in the driver's seat.*

When we arrived at the hospital, there did not appear to be an emergency entrance. We walked into a large square waiting room with signs on the wall admonishing people to be patient. Except for us, the room was empty on a late Friday afternoon. After a short wait, we were taken into an examination room where a kind nurse examined Laurene, and arranged for an X-ray. A friendly doctor prepared a sling for Laurene's arm, gave us a supply of pain meds, and told us to return in three days. The doctor wanted to hear all about our trip. He acted like he hadn't seen anyone in days. He cheered us up, and sent us on our way. We had only been asked to fill out a one-page form with our contact information. No insurance cards, no credit cards, no passport—our first exposure to universal health care.

I contacted the Greenway Hotel and Spa where we had spent the night in Cheltenham. The hotel staff not only extended our stay, but returned us to our same room. Torrential rains followed us back to the hotel. We had difficulty keeping to the narrow roads in the gale, but we managed to get back to the brightly lit manor house. I smelled wood smoke as I parked the car near the front entrance, and walked Laurene into the high-ceilinged entry hall. A bright fire played light on the walls hung with portraits and country landscapes.

In our absence, a hunting party of accountants had arrived from London. They sat around drinking whiskey, smoking pipes and cigars. Everyone looked tweedy in their coats, vests, heavy pants, and high boots. It was like walking into a scene from *Downton Abbey*, including the presence of a yellow Labrador who held down the hearth. Laurene and I were a sorry sight, but we must have been covered with a magical invisibility cloak, because no one noticed us. As soon as we arrived in our room, I removed Laurene's bloodstained clothes, and guided her to the shower. I held her steady while she bathed. She kept apologizing for her fall. She regretted that she would not see the Cornwall Coast.

After the shower and with fresh clothes, we walked downstairs to a parlor where a tuxedoed barman brought us dinner menus and took a drink order. The atmosphere of the formal sitting room gave the happy impression that the world had once been under control, was currently under control, and would evermore continue under control. We were both starved. Laurene was self-conscious about her cuts and bruises, but, as with the hunting party, the reserved guests didn't seem to notice us.

Ever the extrovert, Laurene struck up a conversation with a gray-suited woman in her fifties who sat alone near us, sipping what looked like Campari and soda. The woman told us that she was traveling with a gentleman as his assistant. A few minutes later, a very old man (at least eighty) entered the room as we were called in for dinner. He was nearly bent in half at the waist, wearing a dark pin striped suit and a bow tie. The pair fascinated Laurene, and she entertained me with light-hearted speculation over dinner about the two traveling business companions. By the end of the meal, we had constructed a complete story of their lives. Her medium sherry, pain medication, and the encounter with the unusual couple, combined to take Laurene's mind off her beat-up body.

After eating sea bass in a puff pastry shell, we returned to the room, and I helped Laurene into her pajamas, propped her arm on a pillow, and returned to the bar for an after dinner drink. I savored the events of the day, and looked forward to staying in this 16th century Elizabethan manor house for another three days. The bartender poured me an aged Scottish whiskey—a 12-year-old Balvenie. He lectured me about whiskey, and explained how the alcohol evaporated in the older whiskies, what he called the angel's share. The drink warmed me while I continued to celebrate my momentary gold-star hero status before going to bed.

It rained for the next three days. I purchased some green Wellington boots at a hardware store in town, and took long walks in the rain with an oversized black umbrella, courtesy of the establishment. The manor house took its name from an adjacent, ancient path named GREENWAY. The path led from the house up to the top of a long, high hill. The walking surface rose several feet above the surrounding fields. Half way to the top beside a ramshackle barn, I stopped and looked down on the village and river below. The sun had briefly appeared, and everywhere I looked seemed like an Impressionist painting with vibrant colors pulsing in the soft, moist light.

I wanted to step into the beauty around me, so I climbed over a fence by the path, and walked over to sit on a rock in the middle of a sheep meadow. A few feet from the rock, I noticed the hollowed out stump of an old oak tree. Within the rotting circle of the stump, a slender sapling shot up like an ugly weed. The rotting wood of the fallen tree had nourished the new growth. This observation made me think about how I hardly ever noticed things in detail. Today, it seemed that a different me looked at a world throbbing with radiance. I continued to the top of the hill where I found barrow graves scattered over a prehistoric burial ground that I had been told dated from the Iron Age. Flowers opened in the sunlight.

For three days, I hiked the same path to the top with a knobby walking stick and my new wellies. The images around me sparked my imagination, and as I often did when alone, I began to write a poem on a scrap of hotel note paper. I didn't want to structure the poem in my own way. I borrowed the pattern of the Shakespearean sonnet—three quatrains of alternating rhyme ending in a couplet:

November rains are weeping down the hill,
But I want to brave the stormy gusts this day
To find high ground and watch the Severn River fill.
I walk the stone age path called Greenway.
My Wellingtons trudge up this time-forgotten hill.
Beyond a cowshed, I look down above the village
Shrouded in mist so silvery, silent, and still,
A painting brushed to life from another age.
I sit beside a hollowed stump of tree.
Within the stump's circle, a sapling springs
From the grassy space inside. Now open and free
From the dark soil below, the new growth sings.
Returning down to where I stay,
I find the fiery hearth in the manor of Greenway.

Sipping a Doublewood 12 Balvenie by the fiery hearth after dinner became my nightly ritual— one shot of the old single malt with no ice, to feel its burn down my throat, savor the wood smell, and taste the oak. For a brief time, I felt like Robert Browning who composed these lines while walking through the English countryside over one hundred and fifty years earlier:

The hill-side's dew pearled;
The lark's on the wing;
The snail's on the thorn;
God's in His heaven—
All's right with the world!

Laurene continued her talks with the assistant after breakfast each day, and filled me in on her personal history. The man was a corporate director and widower, and the woman was his personal secretary. The two worked together and traveled together, and the woman, a widow, seemed to be happy with the arrangement, although she might have benefited from the advice of one of Jane Austen's Lady Susan who chided her unhappy friend for marrying an older gentleman who was "too old to be agreeable, and too young to die."

What I enjoyed most about our brief stay at the manor house was the unaccustomed presence of a routine, including the daily appearance of the other lodgers. I realized how unstructured my life had become, and how soothing it felt to know what to expect from one day to the next.

Out of the Inferno

Our last night at Greenway Hotel happened to be November 7, 2000. We watched the U.S. election returns on British television. We went to bed thinking that Al Gore had won. Laurene and I had shared the most intimate conversations on a wide range of subjects, but she had never shared her politics. She had a key that closed the door to her private world, and another one that opened the door. Her politics were behind the closed door. I thought she might like to help elect a native Texan to the Presidency, so she surprised me when she referred to George Bush as a man with a big hat but no cattle. I asked her what she meant. Her comment had nothing to do with George Bush's position on issues. She didn't like how he pretended to be a rancher by burning brush for camera crews.

The next day, we returned to see the jolly English doctor. Even though it was against the rules of the National Health Service, he suggested that we "take a runner" with the X-rays. He wanted our doctor in Houston to see them. He said nothing at the time, but he must have seen bone metastases. The compound break turned out to be more than more than an unintentional injury. The fall had precipitated the break from an arm that had already been weakened by cancer. Now Laurene had metastases in both arms.

The general weakness in her skeleton, particularly in her legs, had most likely caused her to lose her balance while she stood on the stone wall. Her arms would never heal, and other pathological fractures followed.

We returned to London, and stayed a last night at a quaint hotel near the airport. About eight in the evening, I began to swell. My right hand, right arm, neck, and head. I felt my throat tightening. A spider had bitten me earlier in the day causing an allergic reaction. Laurene took immediate action. She struggled to handle the phone with her arm sling. I don't know how she managed to find a local doctor who made house calls, but a doctor appeared at our door within fifteen minutes. He was just as jolly as the doctor in The Cotwolds. After he injected me with an elephant's dose of steroids, the swelling subsided. He stayed in the room to see how I would respond, and when I asked him if he would like a Scotch, he replied, "DON'T MIND IF I DO!"

We flew from Heathrow to Houston the next morning. I had saved Laurene from a Jaguar, and she had saved me from a spider.

LESSON THIRTEEN

Life is either a great adventure or nothing.
—Helen Keller

14.

Leaving the thicket, we came to the border
Between the second circle and the third...
Down every part...a fissure drips tears—
Drip drop drip drop drop drop drop—
Over time, the tears have cut a canyon.

Dante's Inferno, Canto XIV

In 2001, more bones fractured.

Surgeons placed a titanium rod in Laurene's lower left leg, because the slenderest of her long bones had broken. The operation was a success, but an OR technician had misread her chart. The pain meds he ordered for the operation were at a lower dosage than her pain meds had been before the operation. I sat in the waiting room for over twelve hours. No one would tell me what was going on, other than to say that the operation had taken longer than expected.

In the past, the hospital had allowed me to see Laurene in the ICU after an operation. This day, the staff told me to stay in the waiting room. When I finally reached Laurene, she was in bad shape. She told me that her pain level had reached 10 on the 1-10 pain scale, and no one had believed her. She had self-reported using the pain scale for ten years, and in all that time Laurene had never reported more than a 7. She sputtered *"10"* over and over to no avail. After hours of unbearable pain, someone finally checked her chart and adjusted the meds.

We both cried in the ICU. This was the first time in ten years that MD Anderson had let us down. To make matters worse, a physician's assistant arrived and tried to place a blood pressure cuff on Laurene's broken arm. I yelled him out of the room. At that point, she had two broken arms and a broken leg. The assistant returned with a leg cuff for her one good limb. The experiences of this day reinforced for me the need to be with family members during emergency room and hospital stays. The narrow specialties of the staff, the host of electronic monitors, the demands of other patients, all create a ripe environment for missing the changing needs of a single patient.

A few hours later, we landed in a hospital room for the night. I sat in a chair beside Laurene's bed so wound up I couldn't sleep. During the long hours in the waiting room, I had run out of things to do. After finishing two books, and reading magazines that only remotely interested me, I looked around for anything else to read. A large black Bible rested on a coffee table. I turned to Psalms, and started reading familiar passages over and over while daytime television droned in the background. I must have read the 23rd Psalm twenty-five times. Now sitting beside my sleeping wife, I wrote the psalm in my own words:

A Husband's Passage Through Cancerland

God, you care for me.
I don't need a thing.
You lay me down in a grassy meadow.
You lead me by a quiet lake.
You renew my strength
And put my life on a new path.
Even when the way goes through
a valley dark as death,
I'm not afraid when you're around.
Your trusty walking stick keeps me from falling.
You arrange a dinner party for me and invite my enemies—
Not my idea of a good time.
You touch my drooping head
And bless me with extravagant love.
Your goodness and mercy will be there for me
Every day for as long as I live,
Back home in your house forever.

Laurene began physical therapy a few weeks after her leg operation. She loved the therapists. She laughed and joked with them. They seemed to know how to avoid hurting her, even though her mobility had declined significantly. Around the house, she could manage to move stiffly like a broken puppet. I would sometimes move her around the house in a wheel chair. When her hearing began to fail, I would bend over to talk in her ear as I wheeled her along, and sometimes I kissed her behind the ears or on her forehead. I enjoyed making her laugh when laughter didn't hurt. We secretly delighted in a remote ramp at the clinic connecting an old and new building. I would let go of the wheelchair at the top of the ramp, and allow Laurene to go freestyle to the lower level. I always caught the handles to slow her down near the bottom. We laughed like a couple of kids breaking the rules.

Driving from The Woodlands to the clinic one day, a loud pop sounded from Laurene's side of the car. One of her ribs had snapped. I didn't know how to react. Apparently the morphine had masked the pain, because she said, "Oh well, there goes another bone!" Nothing could be done.

I had never imagined this as an outcome of the cancer, my wife breaking into pieces, one piece at at time. The fractures continued. More ribs popped. Her left femur broke next—the largest bone in the body. This time, surgeons inserted a steel rod in her leg rather than a titanium one, using a method called intramedullary nailing. Surgeons inserted the rod into the bone marrow canal to keep her fracture in position, and then screwed the rod to the bone at both ends. When the doctor reported to me in the waiting room, I asked him why steel was used rather than titanium. He told me that steel was less expensive, and Laurene's life expectancy didn't warrant the use of a titanium rod. His cold response took me back.

This operation went more smoothly than the previous one, but Laurene developed sores around the incisions near her pelvis. The sores hurt, and we worried about infection. Too embarrassed to show the doctors, she showed her sores to the nurses. The nurses helped. The nurses always helped.

The latest chemo regimen lost its effectiveness within a few months. Targeted therapies were less developed back then. While we still had treatment options, the choices became increasingly experimental and more limited. In August 2001, Laurene started taking Navelbine. Maybe the cumulative effect of all the chemotherapies together produced the effects, but with this latest drug, all her symptoms worsened: diarrhea, nausea, vomiting, and overall weakness. But she continued with physical therapy. Even though she was dying, physical therapy made her feel better, and she always looked forward to the appointments.

Throughout the year, we made several emergency trips to the hospital when Laurene's pain became intolerable. The ER solution was to shoot her up with steroids. Steroids worked for a few hours, but Laurene had severe withdrawal reactions. She became extremely agitated, and would scream at the top of her lungs. She ripped at her clothes like she had been possessed by a demon. She stood on the furniture.

For all the years of treatment, Laurene had always been calm and rational. I could rely on her to be aware of what was going on. We could talk about next steps and potential problems. Even though she had warned me that she might become ornery, her drug-induced behavior was way beyond ornery. She frightened me. I felt helpless. I called our nurse neighbor. When she arrived, Laurene yelled at her and wanted her to leave the house. This scenario was not a new one for our neighbor. She had handled the situation with others. She hung in there until Laurene exhausted herself, and fell asleep. After the neighbor left, I felt alone and cried. Laurene and I had always been a team.

In October 2001, Laurene underwent a bone marrow aspiration and biopsy. I helped hold her down on a table, while doctors aspirated what they hoped would be healthy marrow to be used in possible future transplants. Nothing stronger than local anesthetic could be used for the procedure. The doctor inserted a large long needle deep into her upper hip to aspirate marrow fluid. Laurene screamed bloody murder. I never got used to her screams. After she caught her breath, he inserted a second needle in the same way to remove bone for a biopsy. She screamed again. A technician placed her bone cells under a microscope. He confirmed that the cancer had spread to the bone marrow.

Laurene developed progressive anemia. She began weekly Procrit injections to build up her red cell counts. The shots gave her headaches, body aches, and more diarrhea. The morphine gave her constipation. We never knew what to expect. I gave her my blood as often as I could (every 56 days). The most serious problem, however, was that blood stream could now carry cancer cells to remote parts of her body, including vital organs.

On the first floor of the clinic, a lab with freestanding wall panels provided people with a convenient place to give blood. One afternoon between Laurene's appointments, I stopped in for another blood donation. I filled out the paperwork, and pulled the donor card out of my wallet. A nurse took my blood pressure. She said that my blood pressure (170/110) was too elevated to donate. I asked her to take a second reading, which confirmed the first. She looked straight in my eyes, and told me that I needed to see a doctor immediately, and that if I experienced certain symptoms like headaches, nausea, vomiting, chest pain, or shortness of breath, I should go to the emergency room.

How could my body be letting me down at a time like this? I thought. I was the strong one. Good health had been a strength all my life. Perfect attendance in school and at work. Laurene was the sick one. I was healthy. She had cancer. I didn't. We were on a parallel journey, but there were differences between us. She was the patient, not me. I was the husband caregiver. Over the next few days, although I didn't have any of the symptoms mentioned by the nurse, I began to feel generally miserable. I didn't feel either strong or good. I felt like I was letting Laurene down, distancing myself from her for reasons I did not understand or even acknowledge.

The following week, my family physician confirmed the high blood pressure, and prescribed blood pressure/diuretic medication. After I gave him an update on Laurene, he suggested that I investigate hospice for Laurene. I resented his suggestion, and told him that Laurene would not need hospice care anytime soon. At the time, however, I regarded hospice as one more thing to do, another hassle. And I wasn't prepared to have the conversation with Laurene. Also, I really didn't know or understand how hospice worked. I imagined hospice as a depressing place that warehoused people, and cut them off from their doctors and other medical care a few days before they died. I could imagine the sign scrawled over the entrance to Hell that had frightened Dante: "YOU, WHO HAVE NO HOPE, ENTER HERE."

My doctor wanted to see me again in a few weeks. He asked me to tell him more about what I was going through with Laurene. I told him that I had trouble sleeping. He offered a sleeping pill prescription, but I declined. Sleeping medication made no practical sense for a 24/7 caregiver. I had to wake up in middle of the night whenever Laurene needed help, and late night trips to the ER happened with increasing frequency. I did fill a prescription for Wellbutrin, an antidepressant. The pills had no effect on me other than a sensation of agitation or edginess, so I stopped taking them.

I talked to a dietician at the clinic, who suggested changes to my diet. The clinic cafeteria offered a wide array of healthy foods, but also lots of highly attractive comfort foods. I had especially loved the breakfast, lunch, and dinner menus at the grill station. I enjoyed standing in line to watch hamburgers sizzle on the grill, and see baskets of fries lifted from the grease pits. Even so, I started going to the salad bar. In addition to eating better, I found time to resume the running routine that I had followed throughout my work career. I lost weight, and when my weight dropped, my blood pressure fell closer to normal.

The cumulative side effects of the successive chemotherapies, radiation treatments, and surgeries added to the burden of the cancer. After ten years of treatment, Laurene's medical file recorded low red and white blood counts, nausea, vomiting, diarrhea, dehydration, constipation, loss of appetite, indigestion, mouth sores, foot sores, dental problems, dry mouth, fluid retention, mood swings, weight loss/gain, arm and leg swelling, osteoporosis, joint pain, slow wound healing, bruising, itching, blistering, insomnia, fatigue, thinking and memory problems (chemo brain), mental disorganization, hair loss, radiation burns, changes in skin color, immobility, peripheral neuropathy, hot flashes, early onset of menopause, and lower sexual desire. I could probably catalog more. And I should add the chaos of anxiety and fear to the top of the list.

On one of our drives home from MD Anderson, we had a typically Laurene discussion about sex. Before and after we were married, no topic had ever been deemed inappropriate. We talked about difficult subjects, no matter how uncomfortable or difficult they happened to be. Laurene talked with the children individually about any and all subjects related to sex and relationships. We also had group discussions in the hilarious setting of family meetings convened by Laurene to discuss household chores, sisterly spats, schedule conflicts...on and on. It took forever to get everyone together in the family room, because no one wanted to be there, except Laurene.

If the family chores weren't getting done, we had a family meeting. If the girls had a fight, we had a family meeting. If family rules (Laurene's rules) had been broken, we all dragged ourselves into the family room for a meeting where the girls sat looking at the ceiling with their arms crossed over their chests. We talked about the importance of grades, study habits, boyfriends and girlfriends, making beds, personal hygiene, health and safety, both weeknight and weekend curfews. During these dreaded meetings, Laurene would cite the misdeeds of other children as learning opportunities for us. Body piercing and tattoos entered the discussions, along with drugs and alcohol. Already little lawyers, the girls had a body of common law precedents from prior cases wherein Laurene, in a weak moment, had relaxed the rules or made exceptions. The girls used Laurene's sense of fairness against her whenever they could to gain an advantage, one of the challenges of having smart children.

So when Laurene brought up the subject of sexuality while driving in the car, I knew we were going to have a "Laurene meeting." She said she was sorry about our lousy sex life. She said that her premature menopause from the chemo and radiation had affected her desire for sex, but more than that, her entire body hurt from bone pain. She thanked me for not pressing her for sex. She told me how much she appreciated her nightly foot massages. We talked about the simple pleasure of being near each other every day. The discussion was short and sweet, like an agenda item in a business meeting. I replied that I didn't love her any less for the absence of sex in our marriage. In perfect irony, our car zipped by a billboard advertising a "gentlemen's club" showing the profile of a young girl with whale-sized breasts sitting on a man's lap.

This turned out to be quite a car trip. Next, Laurene wanted to talk with me about the future.

When I told her in answer to her probes that I had no plans to remarry, she said, "Oh, yes, you will. You're young, and I don't want you to spend the rest of your life alone." In so many words, she told me that I needed someone to take care of me, help me make good decisions, and keep me from getting lost. My limitless capacity to get lost continually amazed her. Over and over, she had explained to me how the exits to parking garages often lead to different streets than the entrance streets. How could I possibly survive on my own?

Then Laurene launched into recommendations for my future partners, accompanied by her evaluation of each one's detailed strengths and weaknesses. The composite of all these women sounded pretty good, but separately I had no interest in any of them. She also listed women who had not made her list and why. In particular, Laurene told me about a woman that I had once said looked beautiful. "She hides varicose veins behind her slacks," Laurene said. "She has the ugliest legs you could ever imagine." From then on, every time I saw the woman in question, I thought about dark purple twisting cords running down her legs. Some of the women on her short list were married. When I said, "What are you mentioning her for...she's married?" Laurene replied that you never know how long a marriage is going to last. I guess she had taken my premarital "no guarantees" speech seriously. I couldn't believe we were having this discussion. Then again, I wasn't surprised.

In the weeks that followed, similar discussions covered wills, personal finances, life insurance, Neil and Stella's farm, Meredith's education, and her own death arrangements. Laurene wanted to be cremated, but she wanted me to ensure that she received a proper cremation. She wanted her ashes to be housed in a sealed blue crystal vase, one of her favorites. She wasn't certain which cemetery she wanted—a plot in Houston where she could be visited more easily, or a plot at the Jordan Springs Cemetery in Brownwood where her grandmother had been buried. She said that she planned to shop cemeteries and would get back to me.

Next, we covered the details of her memorial service. She didn't want the girls to be pressed to speak, so she chose me as the main speaker, along with Sharon, her best childhood girlfriend, and Janet, her bible study leader. The service would be held in the church chapel, not in the sanctuary. She named a soloist, and an organist. She gave me backup names in case one or both of them were not available. When I thought our meeting was over, she said that she wanted me to help her select opening and closing hymns. She only wanted two hymns. So one morning, I opened *The Methodist Hymnal*, and sang over thirty hymns to her. Sometimes, she would sing with me. Other times she asked me to repeat a stanza, or the entire hymn. She finally selected two.

At this time, Laurene decided that it might cheer me up to buy a new car. The odometer on Old Blue, my 1995 Suburban, registered over 160,000 miles. I hadn't been thinking about a new car. When we had bought the car, Laurene's purchasing process had been so excruciating that I never wanted to buy a car again. By now, I had erased Laurene's car buying rules from my mind like a bad memory. As a little girl, Laurene and her father would drive into the country outside of Houston, and shop for cars at small town dealerships. They would trade in the old car, and drive the new one home, but not until they found the right car at the right price. "You always have to walk out at least once," Neil would tell her. She had purchased all our cars since we had been married. Now if I wanted one, I would have to do everything myself, but according to her rules. I decided that I wanted to buy another Suburban in a different color, dark green rather than dark blue.

As I expected, Laurene insisted that I follow the process she had learned from her father. I visited Landmark Chevrolet, and walked out. I visited Courtesy Chevrolet, and walked out. I visited Buckalew Chevrolet, and walked out. I drove to Lawrence Marshall Chevrolet, northwest of Houston. I walked out. The price dropped over $9,000 before I reached a deal with the first dealership that I had visited after they bested the last competitive offer by a mere $150. I hated the negotiations, but Laurene approved. She had passed her father's legacy on to me.

A Husband's Passage Through Cancerland

Laurene liked to give advice to others if asked, however, receiving unsolicited advice from someone else often rubbed her the wrong way. A woman called and said, "Laurene, you shouldn't worry, because you are always safe in God's hands." Laurene did not always feel safe. Her faith in God had ups and downs like the topography of a mountain skyline. There were times when light burned through between peaks like water rushing through an empty riverbed, and other times, when a wall of solid granite blocked all light. Certainly cancer survival had bent her will and tested her faith in every way, as it did mine. She often felt fearful and fragile. Not an intrinsically trusting person, faith came hard for Laurene, and a close relationship with God was not on the top of her list. She wanted nothing more than to return to the life she had. I did, too.

The first thing Laurene asked for during her increasingly frequent visits to the ER was a warm blanket. Blankets weren't always available. Her faith was like that—a warm blanket, but not always available. One night we were lying in bed in the dark.

"My chest feels like a broken cage," Laurene said.

"I'm sorry your ribs are breaking."

"I wish God would open the sky, and give me faith," she said.

"I believe God hears you, and loves you for struggling."

"Do you think so?"

"Yes."

"Why does God want to see me struggle?"

"Because God loves people, and all people struggle. That's what we do."

"You make no sense."

I tried to take another stab at the struggle question, but Laurene had fallen asleep. I was happy to see her sleep, because I had run out of words. Before drifting off, I thought of the lyrics to one of the hymns I had sung for her:

Spirit of God, descend upon my heart.
Wean it from earth, thro' all its pulses move;
Stoop to my weakness, mighty as Thou art,
and make me love Thee as I ought to love.

I ask no dream, no prophet ecstasies.
No sudden rending of the veil of clay,
No angel visitant, no opening skies,
but take the dimness of my soul away.

LESSON FOURTEEN

Faith is fragile.

15.

Now the hardened margin holds us and on we go.
The vapor from the stream forms an overhanging mist
That shields the banks and water from the fire.

Dante's Inferno, Canto XV

2001 PICTURE BOX: last adventures.

Laurene sat by herself at the base of a climbing rock at Garden of the Gods Visitor and Nature Center in Colorado, Springs, the first photograph that I picked out of the 2001 PICTURE BOX, the third and last box. Her smile in the photograph looked forced. I could see the pain in her face. With both of her arms broken, she could no longer take pictures. There were fewer pictures in the third box, more of Laurene and less of me, because I had become the picture taker. We were in Colorado Springs to celebrate my daughter Laura's engagement to Jeremy, her friend since elementary school. They wanted me to experience the top-rope climbing that we had practiced in a gym, outdoors.

While Jeremy and Laura climbed with agility and skill, I felt awkward and heavy. My muscles burned. I wanted to let go, and rest my body. I kept jamming and wedging our fingers, hands, wrists, and arms in cracks, planting my feet on thin crevices, climbing sideways and upwards as best I could, watching my future son-in-law below to hope I'd be caught and held if I fell. Looking back to that year, rock climbing was a metaphor for what Laurene and I experienced. We kept improvising how to keep moving, testing our strength and endurance, depending on others to keep us safe.

2001 was a year filled with lots of activities with family and friends. In June, we rented a large cottage on Walloon Lake in northern Michigan, and invited Jennifer and Meredith's Michigan girlfriends to stay with us—eight in all. The week was organized to celebrate Jennifer's June 2 engagement to Nathan, her boyfriend from Michigan State. Unfortunately, Laurene was in bed most of the time with bone pain. She did manage to visit a bridal salon in Petoskey where Jennifer purchased her wedding dress. I cooked on the outdoor grill, and the girls helped me serve big egg, bacon, and pancake breakfasts, and for dinner, strip steaks, potatoes baked in onions, green salad, and asparagus.

Laurene still managed to take a few snapshots of the girls sleeping. Later it occurred to me that these moments are what we remember most about our children. Not the school photographs or group shots at birthday parties, but a child sleeping, a child crying, a child giggling, a child grabbing your arm for protection after a wet giraffe kiss at the zoo—the best and true maps to the past.

In July, I returned to Colorado Springs to go backpacking with Jeremy and Laura. I needed a break. Laurene encouraged me to go, and made arrangements with her girlfriends to cover for my absence. I drove from Houston to Colorado Springs in one day, and arrived at Laura and Jeremy's apartment late in the evening, in spite of a blowout in Pueblo. After I arrived, we spread our gear on the living room floor. Jeremy removed twenty pounds of stuff from my pack, in some cases, adding some of my weighty items to his own pack. To be left behind: binoculars, flashlight, I would thank him the next day, breathless half way to our 13,000-foot destination.

Early the next morning we drove to Buena Vista, in search of one of the five trails in the Collegiate Peaks Wilderness. We signed in at Browns Pass Hartenstein Lake Trailhead on July 16. I noted that the trail sported a five-star hard rating. We walked six miles up into the lofty statures of mountains amid a world of grasses, sedges, and varieties of wildflowers: Indian paintbrush, blue columbine, alpine sunflower posed for Laura's camera. And wind-blown trees: lodge pole pine, spruce, and fir. We ate wild strawberries along the way. Beauty resided above, below, and around us.

By the time we completed the six-mile segment, we had climbed 1,600 feet. I vowed to never again take any item that was absolutely not essential, which amounted to dry food, water and mosquito repellent. Even my fly rod felt too heavy. We pitched camp by the lake. I looked on in dismay, as Jeremy used my mosquito spray to start the fire. (The mosquito swarms were so think that the sky darkened before sundown.) Jeremy proved to be an expert camp cook. He prepared the perishable food first, and the dried food later. He baked blueberry muffins for breakfast. For snacks, we munched trail mix from a little leather sack, constantly under attack by red squirrels, marmots, and pika. I contributed Mini Oreos, a bag that I had managed to hide when Jeremy plundered my pack.

Jeremy hoisted all the food forty feet over the ground at night. We trekked and fished, and napped in the camp hammock near my tent (one of our few luxuries). We took turns purifying water from the mucky edges of the lake. The lake rested at the bottom of a tree-lined bowl, and one morning, a bull elk appeared to drink in the mist. The elk stood like a statue in the fractured light. The air felt pure. The forest green. The lake blue.

The first night, I heard strange sounds outside my tent. I thought a dangerous animal was about to gnaw through the canvas. I kept looking out of the tent, anticipating an attack, but awestruck by the starshine on the mountains. In the morning, I discovered that the sound was merely a loose tent flap blowing in the mountain wind.

Hungry as bears, we returned to Buena Vista three days later. Lucky for us we pulled into the parking lot of restaurant in Woodland Park with not one, but three huge signs all reading HUNGRY BEAR RESTAURANT. We ordered "nutty bear" pancakes, biscuits and gravy, hash browns, and a "bear" scramble. Each was so huge that it had to be served on a separate plate. On the way home, I wrote this poem:

wild strawberries
in our hands
a perfect tincture
so sweet
we know the savor
of perfection in Nature
at night
above the black angular
shapes of mountains
the Milky Way
radiates splendor
on snow-crusted cirques
as wind scurries to sway
the soft-wooded Ponderosa Tree
we sit
with lips too dry
to utter past or future

*we eat Oreos in silence
and feel free
as flames drop lower
we sleep
renewed, clear
we wake and walk lightly
on the earth
thin in thin air.*

Before Laurene's illness, I hadn't written much of anything since college. Now writing helped me report to myself what was happening to us. Writing, especially poetry, served as a vessel to receive my spilling emotions. Writing filled in the downtime in the waiting rooms, the parts of the day when Laurene slept, the parts of the night when I couldn't sleep. The week after her diagnosis, Laurene had given me a journal with these words handwritten inside the cover:

Dearest Sugar Bear,

Use these pages to express your feelings, list questions, write poetry, whatever helps you with our beat the cancer adventure. I love you very, very much and I am so thankful for your loving support. You're my best friend, and world's best husband.

*Forever,
Laurene*

A Husband's Passage Through Cancerland

On September 11, 2001, I was about to leave the kitchen to help Laurene get showered and dressed for a day of appointments at the clinic. When I glanced at the TV and saw the first plane hit the World Trade Center, I ran into the bedroom to tell Laurene the news. We had no time to watch the news coverage, but we listened to the car radio on our way down Route 45. Laurene hated unneeded deaths. When Princess Diana had been killed in Paris in 1997, she was also very upset. She had tried so hard for so long to keep living, and the fact that either one person or a thousand lost life through senseless war, terrorism, or car accidents was difficult for her to bear. We cried for all the people.

Later in 2001, we went on another family adventure. We drove Jennifer, Nathan, and Meredith from Houston to Brownwood to see the family farm in central Texas. After looping around Austin, Laurene wanted to drive for a change. She said that she could manage the steering wheel underhanded with the range of movement of her least broken arm. She took the driver's seat, and promptly took the speed up beyond 70 mph. At the time, the statewide speed limit was 65 mph after dark. Laurene had always been a fast driver, and had been know to crash a stop sign once or twice. By age five, Meredith had become adept at asking cascades of questions about Laurene's driving habits in perfect imitation of her mother.

"Mom, was that a stop sign back there?"

"Yes, Meredith."

"Mom, aren't you supposed to stop at a stop sign?"

"Yes, Meredith. We are supposed to stop at stop signs?"

"Mom, could you be arrested by a policeman for going through a stop sign?"

"I suppose so...well, yes."

"Mom, could you go to jail?"

Meredith had already mastered her mother's fine art of asking questions.

A State Trooper pulled us over ten miles northwest of Austin. Laurene sweet-talked him out of a ticket by telling him how she wanted to take her children back to see their roots in Brownwood. Maybe he saw her arm sling, and took pity on her. Maybe he recognized that she sounded and talked like he did. In fact, I noticed a subtle change in Laurene's accent as she talked to the trooper. She sounded more Texan than usual.

When we arrived in Brownwood, we picked up Irene Brown, Neil and Stella's friend, who lived on a bluff overlooking a country club where most of the doctors in town lived. The local folks called the bluff "pill hill." Irene was near ninety and badly crippled, but with help from her cook and housekeeper, she fixed us a huge lunch before we set out to find the farm, about five miles outside of town. Irene told us that she would have no problem finding the place. "About five miles down yonder," she said. "Past the cemetery."

When we arrived where Irene directed us, there was a lock on the gate. We had a box of old keys that Neil had left in his garage, but none of them worked. We drove back into town and I bought a bolt breaker at the hardware store. We drove back out to the farm, I busted the heavy chain, and swung the double gate open. We bounced along a dirt road that followed a long rise away from the highway. On the other side of the rise, hundreds of cattle surrounded us. The cattle didn't seem to bother Laurene and Irene, but I had never been on the inside of a fence with what looked up close like big brown monsters. Some had horns. I had no intentions of exiting the car.

Laurene sounded like a character in an old western film, "Someone's been runnin' cattle on Daddy's land!" At home, she didn't drop her "g's," but here she continued to sound like a native Texan. A few minutes later, we drove near the edge of a large, muddy pond (known as a tank in Texas). Irene said, "Neil didn't have a tank near this big."

Out of the Inferno

We had broken into the property next to the Schmitt family farm through the wrong side of a double gate. We had broken a rancher's lock. We had left the gates open. The Brownwood Sheriff's Office had been alerted by a passing pick-up driver. The law was on the way.

Billy Connaway, a distant cousin of Laurene's, appeared out of nowhere riding in a golf cart. He was tall, old, and bent over, similar in appearance to Jack Palance in *City Slickers.* He talked like he was gasping for every breath. He gave me a *not from around here* look. Sensing trouble, Irene Brown took charge. She knew how to handle Texas men. She went on the offensive. Before Billy could open his mouth she said:

Billy, you still seein' that woman down in Brookesmith?

"Yep."

"When are you goin' to marry her?"

"Don't need to marry her," he replied.

"She'd make a fine wife."

"I don't need no wife. I have trouble keepin' a horse."

"*We* think you do," Irene said.

When the matriarch of a large county in central Texas uses the word we, the word has about the same weight as a Supreme Court decision. Billy didn't want to get on the wrong side of Irene, so he decided to be polite. He acted like people broke into his property every day. I happened to notice a shotgun resting to the side of his front door.

Billy had called the sheriff, but when he saw Irene, he knew we weren't cattle thieves. He took us into his house, and showed us a detailed map of the area, including the property lines. He talked about his horses and his cattle and his heart condition, all in the same tone of voice. He offered us iced tea. He spent an hour walking us around, and then we visited the same cemetery Neil had visited on his last day of hunting on his way to breakfast at Irene's place. The Jordan Springs Cemetery had been established in 1887 behind the Friendship Baptist Church. The church had vanished long ago, but the cemetery looked well-maintained. Flowers appeared by many of the gravestones.

Irene Brown managed to hobble over to Laura Schmitt's gravestone. She bent over to read the inscription. The marble gravestone read: Mother, Laura E. Schmitt, March 19, 1889, January 26, 1940. Neil must have paid a lot of money for the gravestone when he had none. It was large by standards of the day, and carved with flowers on either side of "Mother." He had been 29 years old.

In the first half of the twentieth century, women with breast cancer could expect to live three years or less after diagnosis. They endured drastic and disfiguring surgeries, pain, infection, bleeding, and early attempts at radiotherapy. "Mercy, mercy," Irene said. "They burned her up with X rays."

In the fall, I started a new personal adventure—going back to school after thirty years. I enrolled in a statistics course at North Harris College. I thought I might want to go back to school in retirement. Even though I had taken business statistics thirty years earlier at Columbia, I had forgotten most of what I had learned. I also wanted to understand how to interpret the probability and risk factors that I had come across in reading descriptions of Laurene's tests, medications, pathology reports, and clinical trials. As the course progressed, I realized that the study of statistics helped me with my unmet need for order and predictability in the world. The binomial distribution awed me, a family of distributions neither peaked nor flat where the total area under the curve added to 1. As you added additional observations, the distribution approached a normal curve where all the jaggedness of individual observations ended in perfect smoothness.

A Husband's Passage Through Cancerland

The normal curve attracted me by the beauty of its symmetrical shape and its two tails stretching out to infinity in opposite directions. This curve represented a reliable and expression of divine creation in the shape of a bell—the bell curve. Somewhere under that vast curve, all the sampling distributions of all human conditions and forces of nature rested—the healthy and the sick, the good and the bad, the rich and the poor, the survivors and the non-survivors, winds and weather. All the little X-values, like sheep gone astray from the golden mean, followed the summation sign $\sum$ as they imperfectly approached 1. The trajectory of Laurene's disease rested under the tail of the curve in the region of low probabilities, but her condition still resided under the curve, part of the 1.

The rest of the pictures in the 2001 box contained lots of out-of-town visitors: my parents, my brother Dave and his family, old neighbors from Ohio, one of Laurene's classmates from graduate school at Case Western, all of our daughters, including Laura and Jennifer with Jeremy and Nathan, their fiancés. We managed one trip to Cleveland and a trip to Florida to visit my parents, but travel was becoming difficult. Our final trip of the year happened to be the best. Jennifer and Nathan decided to get married in Grand Rapids in December. (Laura and Jeremy set their wedding for June, 2002.)

Out of the Inferno

On the day of Jennifer and Nathan's wedding in Grand Rapids, heavy snow fell all day. A few of the wedding guests from Texas had never seen snow. One of them went out to the rental car lot to see a car blanketed in snow. "Now what do we do?" she said.

Jennifer inherited her mother's skill for organization. The wedding was perfect in every way. Laurene's friends helped dress her, and she looked beautiful. I held her hand while she wept and dabbed her face with a handkerchief in the front row. At the reception, Laurene wanted to dance. She danced until she couldn't move. She didn't want to bring a wheelchair or walker to the reception, so we waited until everyone had left before carrying her out to the car.

LESSON FIFTEEN

Celebrate the temporary!

16.

*I'm leaving behind the bitter and moving toward
   the sweet
Redemption my faithful teacher's promised,
But first I have to reach Hell's lowest level.*

Dante's Inferno, Canto XVI

In January 2002, Laurene and I registered for Spanish classes at the community college. Many of her support people at the clinic were Latina, and she wanted to speak to them in their native language. We sat around long tables with other students, most of whom were fifty years younger than us. Laurene and I enjoyed our studies together, and we tried to speak to each other in Spanish at home and in the car. After a few weeks, we started helping students with their homework. The class was one of the many ways Laurene resisted the disease. "I'm not going to let cancer define my life," she said over and over. Laurene nicknamed me "Alberto," and I called her "Lorena." The experience made me think of my Aunt Alma who had begun piano lessons weeks before she died of breast cancer.

In February, I drove Laurene over to Biloxi, Mississippi to see *Cirque du Soleil*. We had attended a performance in Houston, and Laurene wanted to see another one. The acrobatic company's extraordinary creativity thrilled her. I unloaded the wheelchair, and rolled her through the lobby of a large casino which floated on the Gulf of Mexico. Laurene marveled at the production. Even though her range of movement had become limited, she loved to see how acrobats could twist and turn their bodies to tell a story.

After the show, I asked Laurene if she wanted to gamble. She said that she might want to try a slot machine. I parked her by a quarter slot machine, and told her that I would right back with a ten dollar roll of quarters. "That's too much." She looked around, and spied a garish row of nickel slots. She wanted me to get her a roll of nickels. Three windows showed columns of brightly colored fruit: apples, oranges, cherries, lemons, and watermelons. I moved her to face a nickel machine, and left. When I returned, nickels covered her lap, the wheelchair seat, and had spilled onto the floor. Laurene looked pleased. Three cherries stood in line on the machine.

"Alberto, fantástico! I hit the jackpot. I found a nickel in the bottom of my purse!"

"Wow, what about that?" I said.

"I'm lucky."

"Yes, you are. Want to keep playing?"

"No, we better quit while we're ahead. I'll buy dinner."

Four years later, Hurricane Katrina would hit the casino barge with 55-foot sea waves and push it hundreds of yards inland. Had it survived the storm, the casino would have violated Mississippi's land-based gambling laws. By the time the storm had passed, 166 people were dead, 67 missing, and coastal properties suffered $125 million in damages. Ninety percent of the buildings along the coast were wiped out, including the casino. What are the odds of that? Lower than hitting the jackpot on a nickel slot machine.

In April, the bone metastases had spread to Laurene's head. We looked at the scans on a computer screen. Laurene began radiation treatments to her skull, and the upper extremity of her left arm above the bone shaft and below her neck. With the radiation treatments and bone pain, we had to drop the Spanish course. Since we had neglected to sign up to audit the course, we both received the first failing grades in our academic careers. I read our report cards to Laurene. After all these years, our "permanent records" had been tarnished. The drive to get grades had been so important to us as students, but like so many other things in our lives before the cancer, the need to please others, the need to graduate from a good school, the need to storm the corporate ladder, all these little monsters simply raised up, blinked their eyes, rolled over, and went back to sleep. Nothing mattered more than getting through each day.

One day in June, we had some time in between appointments at the clinic, so we decided to drive over to Rice Village to see a movie. About half-way through the film, Laurene grabbed my arm in the dark theater. Her grip was so tight it hurt me. She had suddenly lost vision in her left eye. She panicked. I loaded her into the car, and drove fast down San Felipe Boulevard, right into a speed trap. A Houston police officer had pointed a radar gun at me, and waved me over to a side street. Laurene opened the passenger door and vomited while the officer wrote the ticket. I tried to explain the circumstances, but he wouldn't listen.

Laurene wanted me to challenge the ticket, so I set up a court date and hired a lawyer. I missed the court day, because Laurene was in the ER. The county issued a warrant for my arrest. So now I had not only flunked Spanish, but I was a wanted man. I was going downhill fast. The lawyer managed to schedule another court date. I sat in a courtroom for the first time. Over the next four hours, I watched how the judge let first offenders off easy, but threw the book at repeaters. When my time came, my lawyer showed the records of Laurene's appointments and the visit to the ER. The judge waived the ticket and fines. Afterwards, she wanted to hear every detail of my court appearance. My getting off assuaged her indignation about the ticket. For me, I simply remember how relaxed I felt spending the day in the air-conditioned court room watching the orderliness of the proceedings and the administration of justice. No one was dying in there.

We soon learned why Laurene had lost vision in her left eye. Tumor cells now pressed against the optic nerve in the back of her eye, and began to paralyze the left side of her face. A few weeks after the incident in the theater, Laurene began to experience episodes of lost consciousness. We met with a neuro oncologist to consider whole brain radiation, a highly controversial procedure. We all decided this was not going to be helpful. The best response would only add another three months to Laurene's life, and the downside effects were formidable: loss of cognition, memory loss, and other brain impairments. After waking from her first episode, Laurene said, *"I've got to get up! I've got to get up!"*

She woke up smiling from another episode and said, "I've just come back from the hallucination station."

"What did you do while you were there?" I said.

"Oh, I talked to God and mother." She gave me this account in a casual way, as if she had just hung up from a phone conversation.

In June, for Father's Day, Laurene surprised me with the most extravagant gift she had ever given me—a Panerai Luminor watch. I had never worn anything more beautiful. Her gifts to me had always been generous, but were usually more practical and much less expensive. A friend must have purchased the watch for her with Laurene's instructions. I later found out that Laurene had managed to get a deal that included a small down payment and zero percent financing. One of her last advices to me was about the watch. "Now don't you pay it off early," she said.

On an early autumn morning in 2002, Laurene recovered from another episode of unconsciousness. "What's on the agenda today?" she said.

"What would you like to do?"

"I want to go Christmas shopping for the girls. I may not live until Christmas."

"You might kill yourself shopping."

"What do I have to lose?"

These days getting Laurene ready to go anywhere took the better part of two hours—eating, taking medicine, bathing, dressing, applying ointments and make-up, and finding the silicone boob to insert in a pocket of her bra. The boob always seemed to be misplaced. When we were about ready, we double-checked for what we needed to bring along: purse, sunglasses, bottled water and snacks, medications, sunglasses, a cushion for the wheelchair, plastic grocery bags, and extra clothes for emergencies.

Late morning, I adjusted the leg rests on the wheelchair, moved Laurene from the bed to the chair, and wheeled her to the front door. I backed the car out of the garage. On this day, three of our four daughters were with us, so the girls and I managed to lift both Laurene in the wheelchair from the threshold of our front door down two steps to the level of our front walk. I eased Laurene into the front seat. After folding up the wheelchair, and loading it into the trunk, we backed out of the driveway for our adventurous shopping trip. I drove slowly out of the neighborhood, and took my time with turns. Impatient drivers honked, but we were all in a great mood, and the day was sunny and beautiful.

The traffic on our way to the Galleria was heavier than usual. As we approached the Route 290 junction, Laurene said, "Everybody and their dog is out today!" At that moment, we heard honking horns and screeching brakes. A dog was crossing twelve lanes of traffic on either side of the crowded freeway. We rooted for the dog who darted and dodged like a professional half back through the scrimmage of cars and trucks. We cheered when he made it to the other side, then we laughed ourselves silly. *"Everybody and their dog is out today!"* we all said in chorus.

On October 7, Laurene's doctor wrote this clinic note: "The patient reports that she would just like to feel possibly a little better." Never a complainer, Laurene perpetually understated her condition, even when talking to her doctor.

The Procrit shots to maintain Laurene's blood and platelet counts became less effective, and so beginning in October, she began to receive weekly blood transfusions. I gave blood and plasma as often as I could. She continued physical therapy until late October when shortness of breath ruled out further sessions. Cancer had spread to the lining of her lungs. A doctor effused malignant fluid from her lung cavity. About this time, her right clavicle fractured, and a special sling held her shoulder blade in place. Nausea and vomiting increased. During this time, we drew closer to each other. Rather than resisting or distancing ourselves from suffering, we let the suffering embrace us. We had run out of places to go and things to do. We had run out of adventures. Falling back on ourselves, we engaged in quiet conversations, and managed to enjoy Laurene's increasingly infrequent pain-free moments. The days stretched out to last lifetimes.

During these last days, Laurene wanted to talk about my future. Now that she had no future, she wanted to focus on mine. I told her that I had no desire to go back to work for a large corporation, and that I had altogether lost my interest in business. She thought that my interest in college teaching would be a good idea. She kept bringing up the topic, and wanted to know how I could get ready for this new career. With her encouragement, I purchased prep books and began to study for the Graduate Record Exam. I hadn't taken a standardized test for over thirty years.

With a "you can do it!" cheer from Laurene, I took the GRE at the University of Houston. I scored well enough to qualify for entry into all but the most elite doctoral programs. The low score on spatial reasoning did not surprise me, since I have never done well mentally manipulating objects in my mind, and I've spent most of my life getting lost while trying to follow a map. During the test, a monitor embarrassed me when she walked by and observed me trying to measure the sides of isosceles triangles and trapezoids by pressing the edge of my scrap paper against the computer screen. When I showed Laurene my test results, she said, "I knew you would do well. You have a good brain. That's one reason I decided to marry you."

Laurene's pain level kept getting worse, so we made an appointment at the Pain Management Center at MD Anderson. The doctor prescribed oral doses of patient-controlled morphine (too little, you have unacceptable pain relief; too much, you drop into a coma or die). Laurene liked the idea of having control over her pain. With the addition of the morphine, I now had a lengthy spreadsheet of her medications organized by type, dosage, and frequency. I spent 30-45 minutes a day to plan the medications, and to maintain the supply line of prescriptions. Laurene worried about addiction. She didn't want to become an addict. The doctor assured her that she needed the morphine, and that she would not become a drug addict.

About this time, Laurene's brain began to swell further, paralyzing the left side of her face. Bone metastases had spread to her pelvis. At bedtime each night, I massaged her feet with peppermint lotion. As I lay down to sleep, I worried that she might slip away in the night, swept away the unbridled advance of the cancer cells. Hope had no future.

Even though Laurene expressed concerns about my future, she still had unfinished work of her own. Our shared office was right near the bedroom. One day I noticed Laurene's handwriting on a scrap of paper. She wrote: "My life is releasing joy." I knew at that moment that she had found a place on the other side of her suffering. Like Dante, she was "moving on from the bitter to the sweet."

From this sweet place, she began to compose letters. She started writing to Meredith and Jennifer.

A Husband's Passage Through Cancerland

She drafted the letters over and over again. She would print them out, read me excerpts, then throw the drafts away and start new ones. After she finished writing to her daughters, she began letters to my daughters. She never finished. She tried to write a letter to me, but she couldn't. She told me that she had tried, but she couldn't write another word.

"You don't need to," I said. "We all know you love us...and we all love you."

LESSON SIXTEEN

Keep one foot in this world when the other one is in the next.

17.

So I went on alone even farther along
The outer margin of the seventh layer
To where the sufferers were sitting.

Dante's Inferno, Canto XVII

By the first week in November, Laurene was attached to oxygen and could no longer walk. Rather than weekly red blood cell and platelet transfusions, she now received two infusions a week. Her blood counts kept dropping. At the end of one of the transfusions, her doctor entered the room. He said that the frequency of the transfusions would keep increasing, and that the benefit of more transfusions would most likely be outweighed by the risks of immune reactions, fevers and chills, and other complications. He told her that she should consider hospice. He left the hospital room, and said he would come back to see what we decided. It was time for our toughest decision. We discussed how the hardest part would be cutting the umbilical cord to the doctor and clinic that had kept her alive for over eleven years.

When the doctor returned, Laurene thanked him for serving as her advocate for so long. She agreed to hospice, but wanted to know if she could still contact him if she needed to. He agreed. Then he bent over her, and kissed her. When he reached the door, he stopped. He turned around and looked at Laurene. I thought he had something more to say. Then he turned back around, and gently closed the door. We stared at the closed door. The doctor was gone. Until that moment, I had never realized how hard it must have been for him to stand by us through all those years, maintaining his professional demeanor, keeping his passion for curing cancer and teaching others, using his intelligence, charm, and wit to keep Laurene's hope alive—and all the time, holding the burden of concern and knowledge about Laurene's condition.

"Did you see that! He turned around to see me again! He's going to miss me!" Laurene said. We both loved him. When the door closed, we felt like the air had been sucked out of the room.

Laurene shopped hospices in the same way that she purchased cars. She invited three hospice reps to the house for presentations. She asked her "Laurene" questions. She asked me to do reference checks. A week later, we picked the one that seemed the most flexible.

On November 7, we set up hospice in our bedroom. Hospice staff arrived with equipment, medications, supplies, and a raft of consent forms. We set up oxygen tanks with lines running from one end of the house to the other, and placed a hospital bed next to our bed. The nurse told me to buy dark-colored sheets and blankets for the bed so they wouldn't show stains.

By the time the hospice doctor arrived for her first visit, Laurene had dropped into a coma. I was standing on one side of the bed, and the doctor stood on the other side. She asked me to review Laurene's medical history. I recited the names and sequences of all the chemotherapies, radiation treatments, and surgeries. In the middle of my recitation, Laurene emerged from her coma, and tried to raise herself up to speak. She wanted to correct me, but she couldn't produce the words. The doctor gently lowered Laurene back down on the bed, and assured her that she had enough information. In a way, I was glad this happened. It meant that Laurene could hear us—even from a coma. But I had better keep my facts straight.

After the doctor left and the nurses had finished their daily visit, I felt overwhelmed by the responsibility of caring for Laurene alone under the present conditions. If trouble occurred, I couldn't merely step out of the room and yell for a nurse like I had done in the clinic or hospital. As I stood beside the hospital bed looking down at Laurene, she opened her eyes. She was trying to speak again. She managed to whisper, "I can't breathe." As I turned to run for the phone, I noticed that I had been standing on the oxygen line. Hospice had only been established in our home a few hours, and once again, I had screwed up.

Laurene went back to sleep. *An easy fix. Don't stand on the oxygen lines.*

A few days later, Laura and Jennifer arrived. Laura stayed for a weekend. The presence of the girls enlivened Laurene, and she woke up. Laurene asked me to get her out of bed and wheel her into the kitchen where she could meet with Laura in private. Afterwards, Laura told me that the meeting was very difficult for her. She felt shy and awkward. She really didn't understand the purpose of the meeting, until Laurene told her that she hoped Laura knew she loved her. Laura replied that she knew Laurene loved her, and she said that she loved Laurene, too. They both cried, and then hugged. Laura said she felt hot and uncomfortable after the meeting. She went upstairs and cried some more. Years later, Laura told me that having the talk with Laurene meant more to her than any words that were exchanged, the notion that Laurene wanted to include Laura in her farewells.

After seeing how fast Laurene was failing, Laura flew back to Colorado, requested a leave from her teaching job, and completed lesson plans through Thanksgiving. She returned a week later. The week of November 10, Meredith arrived. Laurene had wanted Meredith to finish her semester at Vanderbilt. It's hard for me to describe how relieved I was to have my beautiful daughters in the house. I felt supported and loved. The girls fixed meals, and helped take care of Laurene. Jennifer helped me figure out the schedule of medications. Laura and Jennifer rolled Laurene over so I could insert suppositories. The girls added a lightness to the house—banter, laughter, joy—and everyone taking care of each other the way families do.

Nathan, my new son-in-law, helped me move Laurene outside to our back porch on a sunny afternoon. She wanted to see the pool and the gardens, and watch the birds and squirrels. Later, she asked Nathan to bring her favorite painting into the bedroom, a bright palette knife painting of Positano, a cliffside village on southern Italy's Amalfi Coast. Nathan removed the painting from the fireplace mantle in the family room, and held it at the foot of the hospital bed. He entertained her by clowning around. He disappeared behind the painting, and then popped his grinning face out from each side. He brought joyful tears to her eyes. From the first time she had met Nathan, Jennifer had called him, "Mr. Fun."

The girls helped me manage the visitors. One day, a woman who lived nearby paid a visit. "We're praying for you every day," she said. "You just have to have a more positive attitude, and Jesus will make you well." The woman vanished. She was there, and then she wasn't. I think Jennifer must have escorted her out of the house so fast that the lady's feet didn't touch the ground. Like her mother, Jennifer always took charge when the occasion required. The first time I stood on the front porch of Laurene's house to take her on a date, Meredith had opened the door. She was five years old with long blond hair, and it was obvious that Laurene had dressed her up to make a good impression.

"Are you going to be my new daddy?" she said.

Jennifer appeared out of nowhere, looking up at the sky in disgust. She put one arm around her little sister's neck, and dragged her out of sight like a marionette on a play stage. I'm pretty sure she did the same thing with the neighbor lady.

Visitors kept coming to see Laurene, and I don't know why, but everyone wanted to touch her. They felt bad when Laurene yelped with pain, but it was too late. We soon established "do not squeeze" ground rules for the visitors, and limited their visits to no more than fifteen minutes. At night, Jennifer and Laura slept in the bedroom on our bed, next to the hospital bed. I either slept on a sofa in the bedroom, or in the downstairs guest room on the other side of the house.

When Laurene and I were alone, we had short conversations, but she kept slipping out of consciousness. I never knew when she would wake up, so we all took turns sitting by the bed. I set up a baby monitor for the times she was alone in the bedroom. Even with the girls' help, I was getting tired. Everyone was tired. About a week after we set up hospice, Laurene began fecal vomiting. Fortunately, the hospice nurse was with me when this first happened. "Her liver's shutting down," she said. One of the most resilient organs in the body, the liver had finally succumbed to the cancer.

Managing the morphine proved to be difficult. We didn't want to kill Laurene with an overdose, but we didn't want her to suffer either. I hadn't realized that the range of medications provided by hospice had placed me in the position of making life or death decisions. Half the time, Laurene lay in a semi-conscious state, and half the time she experienced extreme pain. There seemed to be no middle place. One afternoon, Laurene woke up, and called out one word repeatedly. We finally figured out that she was saying, *"back...back...back."* A Beanie Baby that the girls had placed on her shoulder had fallen behind her back. It's lumpy little body jabbed her. When we removed the toy, Laurene closed her eyes and gave us a faint smile of relief, the same smile I had received after restoring her oxygen supply.

While Laurene wanted to die at home, I'm not sure hospice in the home worked for us. While home hospice gave us more access to Laurene, we were getting burned out. Also, Laurene needed 24-hour skilled nursing, and we couldn't give her all of the professional care she needed. When she was conscious, Laurene bundled her requests to be easy on us. She would ask for us to change her position in bed, give her a drink of water, or ask us to help move her to the potty chair.

One evening while I was bathing her in bed, she said, "What's happening to me?"

"You're dying with dignity," I said.

"I'm afraid to die," she replied.

I've thought about her words for a long time. I don't think Laurene was spiritually unprepared for death, but the thought of stepping into the unknown frightened her. Who would not be afraid? Christ was afraid when he called out, *"Why hast thou forsaken me?"*

Right before death the stakes are raised horribly high. The most well-grounded beliefs are tested—even more when suffering has knocked you down over and over. I had to think, *would my own beliefs about eternal life fall like a house of cards in the face of imminent death? Would my faith even survive bouts of intense physical pain, let alone dying?*

I also thought about how brief our conversations had been near the end. There had been no idyllic death scene where we said goodbye and wrapped up unresolved issues, forgave each other for crimes and misdemeanors, made promises, and received last advices. The drugs, the pain, the frequent losses of consciousness all contributed.

I comforted myself with the thought that during all those trips to and from MD Anderson over all those years, and from a lifetime's worth of conversations with the girls, everything that we had to say had been said.

LESSON SEVENTEEN

Satisfying endings are rare. Death happens in the same way that life happens—loose strings with frayed ends.

18.

With that, I think we've seen enough.

Dante's Inferno, Canto XVIII

On the evening of November 16, 2002, Laurene had slipped into another coma. Jennifer and Laura slept together in our bed next to the hospital bed. I slept in the guest room at the other end of the house. About four the next morning, Laura walked into my room to tell me that Laurene's breathing had changed. Laura first noticed the change a half hour earlier, and had alerted Jennifer. They listened to Laurene's breathing—the intervals between breaths kept getting longer, so they decided to wake me.

In the bedroom, I lay my head down on the flat, scarred side of my wife's chest, facing the slope of her one good breast. I listened there for her heart, but could only hear and feel my own heart. She had died. She had a faint smile on her face like a good-natured traveler who had come home after covering a vast territory—eleven years battling breast cancer. With all the medical advances since the 1940s, she had only lived a few years longer than her grandmother.

I hugged her hard. I no longer had to worry about hurting her broken bones. We all wept over the spent body that no longer housed her. I left the bedroom and called hospice. A hospice nurse arrived in twenty minutes, and began to prepare the body for transportation. She placed a rolled up towel under Laurene's chin so her head wouldn't fall to one side. I stayed with Laurene, and reflexively rubbed her feet with peppermint lotion. Her long body lay flat on the bed like a map of pain and sorrow. Her body would no longer be cut and squeezed and poked and filled with poisonous fluids. I looked at her face. The pain and the fear and the worries were gone. I stood by her bed for a long time.

Darkness passed to semi-dark dawn to the bedroom's white quiet. The room seemed colorless. I hadn't expected Laurene to die this particular night. I knew she was near death, but I had thought she would live for a few more days or even weeks. Now it seemed like she had packed up and slipped away unannounced in the middle of the night. So unlike her.

I looked at her ridges of scars and radiation burns. Laurene's body looked like a battlefield. At that moment, I realized that the cancer survivors' metaphor of a cancer journey didn't match what I observed at the moment, or over the survival years. I may have been on a journey, but she had been at war. For the first time, I accepted why the obituaries often read *she died after a long battle.* It truly had been a battle all along. Journey might describe the experience of breast cancer survivorship in part, but for the dead, battle best describes what I witnessed before me. She had been a warrior. She had *fought the good fight, beaten the odds. She had outlived the survival estimates. She had lived for years under the tail end of the survival curve.* I looked down at my new watch for the time, the last gift from my wife.

At 6:00 AM on November 17, 2002, the hospice doctor pronounced Laurene dead. Her death certificate read: *Laurene Lucille Evans, Schmitt (maiden), November 17, 2002, Date of Birth, February 18, 1947, Hispanic Origin, No, US Armed Forces, No, Education, 17+ years, Marital Status, Married, Surviving Spouse, Albert Randall Evans, Jr., Usual Occupation, Teacher, Kind of Business, Public Education, Father's Name, Neil William Schmitt, Mother's Maid Name, Stella Mae Rice, County of Death, Montgomery, Precinct #3, Place of Deposition, Brookside Crematory, Funeral Home, Forest Park The Woodlands, Immediate Cause, Invasive Ductal Carcinoma of Breast with Metastasis, Interval Between Onset and Death, 11 years. Autopsy, No, Did Tobacco Use Contribute to Death? No. Registrar File No. 01-1495-02. Date Received by Local Registrar, November 19, 2002.*

After the doctor left, a hearse arrived from the funeral home. We had dressed Laurene in her favorite Shepherds of Australia dress and a colorful head scarf. We all cheered as they wheeled her away. Cried and cheered at the same time. The hospice nurse asked me to sign a form and hand over the medications. All that was left were the oxygen tanks, the wheel chair and walker, the potty chair, and the hospital bed. I wheeled the hospital bed out of the bedroom, and removed all the equipment to another room. The hospice nurse stripped the bed, and removed the medications. She gave me a form to sign, then left.

The battle image kept repeating in my mind. She had won the battle. She had won the battle. Every cancer cell was now dead, and she's still around somewhere, maybe having a party in Heaven with Neil and Stella. No more pain. Now what? What about me? What's next for me?

By 7:00 AM, Laurene's body had left the house. I had known she was going to die for a long time, but I felt like she had left suddenly and without a proper goody-bye, without one of her thank you notes, and without an annotated list of her rules to live by. I felt like she had been hit by a car. There was an unfathomable emptiness ahead, like I had been shot into space. I had a whole day staring at me. I needed to do something. I called the church and the funeral home. The girls and I tackled the long contact list. I called the medical equipment company. I wanted all that stuff out of our home, my home.

We started working on the obituary and the memorial service. I don't remember if we ate breakfast or lunch, but in the early afternoon, I dropped into a lounge chair on the back porch by the pool. Not more than several hours after Laurene's death, I decided to break one of her rules. I clipped the end of a thick dark cigar and struck a match. As the blue smoke began to rise, Jennifer appeared from inside the house. "Mom told you not to smoke." I don't think Jennifer objected to the cigar as much as what it represented—a change to a new family system not necessarily governed by her mother's rules; a world other than her mother's where she was already feeling less protected and secure.

The next day, we started going through Laurene's things. She had left what she called her rat piles throughout the house. She had told me how embarrassed she was about leaving work for everyone. She never threw anything away, a habit that she had inherited from Neil and Stella who had learned their lessons of economy from the Great Depression. In the middle of all this, one of the kids called out from Laurene's closet. We all walked to the closet where Meredith stood holding a fistful of twenty dollar bills. Laurene had planted cash in socks, hats, beneath lingerie, stuffed into off season clothes, in between piles of papers, in drawers and on shelves throughout the house. I'm certain that she had planned her surprises to reward us for cleaning up her rat piles.

By the time we were finished, we had over $3,000 in cash that she must have squirreled away months before when she could still walk. Our work did not result in a neat home, but rather an empty house. Each item packed away or disposed of was like a memory deleted, gone. Thousands of memories attached to hundreds of familiar objects, gone. Gone were the hand-written notes about everyday matters, gone the piles of unread books and magazines, gone the cosmetics (the girls and I each saved a small bottle of her perfume, Estee Lauder Youth Dew), gone her calendar. We saved Laurene's best clothes for her girlfriends to try on after the memorial service. Some would go to the Women's Resource Center. The rest to a consignment store.

The funeral director let us visit Laurene in her brown plywood casket before the transfer to the crematorium. She looked peaceful and natural even though she was dead. Laurene had given me specific instructions about her cremation before she died. She had read about the discovery of 334 unidentified bodies at Tri-State Crematory near Chattanooga, stacked in vaults, tossed in buildings, thrown in holes, and cast in woods. So she wanted me to follow her body to the crematorium to make sure everything happened properly. She didn't want to be lying somewhere out in the open like a thrown away corpse in a Stephen King novel.

Jeremy and I followed the hearse to an unfamiliar part of town near a freeway. We entered the building, and I asked the attendants to open the casket once again. Yep, she was there. After the lid was replaced, I bent over the wooden box and prayed.

A Husband's Passage Through Cancerland

The huge retort was already fired up. The attendants placed the casket on roller bars, opened the furnace with a red button, and pushed the casket into the glowing orange furnace. I wanted out fast. Most people experience cremation as paperwork, filling out forms, following a procedure, an affordable alternative to body burial, environmentally friendly.

I stood in the parking lot and watched white smoke gust out of the chimney. There was a rising of wind in the trees, and the smoke dissipated and blended into the morning air. Traffic rushed on nearby. My wife's body had gone up in smoke. Out of the inferno. I wanted to believe in eternal life, but at that moment, Laurene seemed no less dead than the leaves around my feet.

LESSON EIGHTEEN

Death of a loved one comes as if a new season has arrived—abruptly. You think you might have a long autumn full of color, and the next day the temperature drops forty degrees, the leaves fall from the trees, and the ground freezes.

19.

It was here he gently set his cargo down—

Dante's Inferno, Canto XIX

The morning after Laurene's death did not go as I had expected. It was a noisy, sad morning, which disappointed everyone in the house. I planned to cook a full breakfast for the girls, and then, I thought that we would sit around the table to chat and plan the activities of the day. I screwed up the breakfast. People kept calling for details, delivery men knocked on the door with flowers, a medical supply truck arrived to pick up the oxygen tanks. With all the flurry, I overcooked the scrambled eggs and undercooked the bacon. The girls moved little rubbery egg balls around their plates like yellow turds. I burned the toast and we had no butter.

Then if a bad breakfast hadn't been sufficient to start the day off wrong, the girls started to squabble. Her older sisters went after Meredith for some snarky remark she had made. Laurene had always protected Meredith as the youngest. I choked down my eggs while the fight continued. Jennifer began to lecture Meredith about her bad behavior. Meredith interrupted with a heart-felt response:

"I need you to be my sister, not my mother!"

As we cleared the breakfast disaster area, I thought about what Meredith had said. *If Meredith doesn't want her sister to become her mother, then the girls probably don't want me to become their mother either. I need to be the best possible father, especially now, but I shouldn't try to replace Laurene, not that I could if I tried.*

For me, a larger problem loomed. How was I to replace everything that Laurene had done for me throughout our marriage? She had only let go of her duties when she could no longer perform them because of the cancer. For example, when the girls got into fights, I would watch as a bemused bystander while Laurene sorted things out. She had also planned our social life and our vacations. She had communicated with our parents and other relatives. She had handled everything related to our household. Since I was notoriously unhandy, she had an address book filled with people who could fix about anything that broke. Other than writing the bills each month, I hadn't needed to lift a finger to live a comfortable life. While Laurene asked my opinion about matters, she mostly reported how she had solved problems.

If Laurene had been around the morning after her death, she would have fixed breakfast, settled their arguments, called friends and relatives about her death, sent her obituary to the newspapers, and set plans in motion for her memorial service. She would have provided instructions for flower arrangements, and recommended charitable organizations for donations on her behalf, along with addresses and phone numbers. She would have told the girls what clothes to wear for her service. She would have comforted each of us according to our needs, seeking to heal our wounds—the physical, mental, and emotional wear and tear that her passing had caused.

So, I felt irritated. I would have to fill the gaps created by Laurene's departure. In so many areas of our life, I had been the second or third string bench sitter, an amused spectator who followed the game from the safety and comfort of the sidelines. I had enjoyed the many benefits of having married a smart, strong woman, but now my string had run out. I stared at her empty, folded-up wheelchair.

My familiar world had disappeared, and had been replaced with a new strange one. Even though all the bedrooms were full, the house seemed empty. The neighborhood took on the unusual, weird look of a foreign country. The weather had changed from warm fall to cold winter. Beneath my surface feelings, fear tapped against my head like a ball-peen hammer. In *Grief Observed,* C. S. Lewis wrote: "No one ever told me that grief felt so like fear."

Even though we had not communicated much in her last days, I missed Laurene's daily presence more than anything. She had disappeared below the surface of my everyday life. I felt like I was swimming under water looking up for a light distorted by the water. I felt disoriented, saddened, but these emotions layered over the deeper emotion of fear, not fear of the unknown, as much as fear of abandonment.

But we had a lot to do. We all wanted to do a good job on the memorial service, something that Laurene would expect. She had died on the Sunday before Thanksgiving week. To make it easier for the out of town people who would be coming, we planned to hold off on the service until the Saturday following Thanksgiving weekend. The girls stayed with me at home, and within a few days, my parents arrived from Florida. My brother and his family arrived from Atlanta a few days ahead of the service. Friends flew in from around the country. The girls helped me book flights and hotels, organize the memorial service, make final arrangements with the funeral home, place the obituaries, book an organist and soloist, meet with the pastor, and cook meals. They went shopping for colorful outfits to wear to the memorial service, a tribute to their mother's love of color.

The problem with all this was that I didn't want to talk to all these people outside the inner circle of my immediate family. I knew I had to be available to everyone, but I didn't have time to be alone, to figure things out, to decide what to do after everyone left.

The time between Laurene's death and the memorial service proved difficult. I kept telling people that I had "lost" my wife, as if she had disappeared, but could still be found. My house seemed empty and hollow, even though all the bedrooms were full. All of the rooms seemed too big, and filled with harsh light. Laurene's dog-eared address book sat on the kitchen counter, not where it belonged by the phone in the office. Her familiar rat piles of notes and turn-out magazine pages had been removed. The place looked too tidy. The trunks of the Yaupon trees lining the backyard pool appeared contorted, and the leathery, brown leaves looked sparse, and the twigs no longer held birds. The once-abundant flower beds had wintered themselves into the ground. Nothing looked the same. The house and neighborhood was devolving into the anonymity of any other house and any other neighborhood, from abundant colors to dull, reddish-brown sepia tones.

One afternoon that week, I walked down the street of my once-familiar neighborhood to the row of mailboxes. I stood by the mailbox and shuffled envelopes. There were tons of sympathy cards, hospital bills, a contract from the funeral home, and a flyer addressed to Laurene that offered a free mammogram.

A young boy in the neighborhood walked up to me. I could hear the flap of his flip flops on the pavement. Some months earlier, he had come over to my side yard while I was cleaning a catch of white bass from Lake Conroe. I taught him how to debone fish without cutting himself. We had a good time. I don't remember his name, but he was a friendly little boy, about nine.

"Did you hear? Some lady in the neighborhood died. My mom said they drove her away in the back of a big black car," he said.

"My wife," I replied.

"Sorry." He walked away red-faced.

I wish the process of grieving could be as uncomplicated as this conversation the boy. I heard your wife died. Yes, she's dead. Sorry.

Laurene had not only told me who she wanted to speak at the memorial service, but who she did not want to speak. She didn't want anything too emotional or long-winded or overly preachy. She had requested short speeches from Sharon, her best friend, from Janet, the leader of the women's bible study group, and from me. So I had known far in advance that I would not be able to sit silently with my girls in the front row while dabbing my face with a white handkerchief. Laurene had told me that we three were the only people she trusted to do a good job of sending her off. Writing what I would say was probably as difficult as the letter Laurene had wanted to write to me, but could not. What would honor her best? Should I use humor? What if I started to cry? And if I started to cry, could I stop and go on?

On the day Laurene died, I had followed my usual routine by picking up a copy of *The New York Times*. Every Monday morning during the first semester of my freshman year at Ohio University, my government professor had quizzed us on *The Week in Review*, so I had been reading the *Sunday Times* since 1968. I wasn't ready to write my remarks for the memorial service, so I picked up the paper to see what news happened on the day Laurene died. A delaying tactic.

Some of the stories: *Barry Bonds wins fifth National League Most Valuable Player Award, Lleyton Hewitt beat Roger Federer to reach the final of the season-ending Masters Cup in Shanghai, Columbia loses to Cornell 17-14 in seven straight losses, President Vicente Fox of Mexico hints that he would not support the US resolution threatening Iraq in the United Nations, JFK medical files reveal a hidden illness, Send in No Clones, the challenge for bioethics, Nancy Pelosi assumes leadership of House Democrats, the Bush administration proposes to keep snowmobiles in Yellowstone, Navy to limit sonar testing thought to hurt sea mammals, famine threatens 15 million people in Ethiopia. Abba Eben, South African-Israeli soldier and politician dies (b. 1915), Frank McCarthy, American painter and illustrator dies (b. 1924).*

The long lives of Eben and McCarthy prompted me to think about what more Laurene might have accomplished had she lived another twenty or thirty years. Before her diagnosis, Laurene had been invited to Croton, Connecticut to meet Jack Welsh, then CEO of General Electric. GE Lighting had supported her inclusion in this elite group of high-potential employees. Perhaps she might have become GE's CEO one day. Maybe she would have gone back to school to become a lawyer, her childhood dream. Maybe she would have returned to teaching, her first job out of college. *Death matters,* I thought. *Death has permanent consequences. Lost opportunities for both career and family. Laurene would never live to retire with me. She would not know her grandchildren.*

On November 20, the girls took me out to dinner for my 56th birthday. We had a good time talking, and the kids showered me with fun gifts. Mom and Dad stayed through Thanksgiving, and the family of Meredith's best friend invited us to their home for Thanksgiving dinner. At the house, Mom made sugar cookies and pecan pies. I drove Mom and Dad into the country around Brennan. Laura and Amy flew back to Cleveland for Thanksgiving with their mother, and then returned the day before the memorial service on Saturday, November 30.

We held the memorial service in the chapel of The Woodlands Methodist Church. With a 300-seat capacity, mourners filled half the chapel. I sat in the first row with the girls. A single photograph of Laurene sat on a small table before the altar. Sprays of flowers stood on either side. When it was my turn to speak, I looked out over the people sitting there. Friends, family, neighbors, women from Rosebuds, people from church, nurses from MD Anderson, former business associates, Neil and Stella's friends and family, Laurene's classmates from high school and college, including a few of her Delta Zeta sorority sisters. Mercedes, our housekeeper who had become a US citizen with coaching from Laurene, sat in a pew with her girlfriend. Out-of-town friends attended from half a dozen states.

The opening prayers, the music, and the scripture readings gave me hope that the service would take on the comforting familiarity of a church service. We sang the hymns Laurene had chosen. When my turn came, I didn't want to leave the pew. I had underestimated the difficulty of speaking at my wife's memorial service. I feared that I would break down, and start crying nonstop. My hands were shaking, and my feet felt so heavy that I thought they might sink into the marble floor.

I found a few familiar eyes in the pews, and directed my words to them. I found that I could talk through eyes blurred with tears. I thought about how Laurene would say to the girls and me, *"Keep breathing...you can do it!"* I had written two pages, and looked down to find the neatly printed words that described two or three imperfect anecdotes that would have to serve as a way to sum up Laurene's life. I wanted to say, "These stories are just examples. Laurene's life was so much more than what I've told you."

But I heard Laurene say, "No, no, don't do that." So I didn't.

As the service ended and organ music played, I walked down the aisle with John. Each of us had been married to the same woman for fifteen years. "We were both lucky," I said.

"Yes, we were," he replied.

A few days later, we all gathered at the memorial park to place the blue crystal vase with Laurene's ashes in a niche. We formed a circle, held hands, and said a prayer. Mosquitoes began to eat us alive. Under her name, the plaque read, OUR BLUEBONNET ANGEL. Every time I revisited the memorial park over the next several months, fresh flowers had been placed beneath her marker. I wasn't the only one who grieved her passing, and was trying to live in a world without her.

Laurene had been dying for a long time, and I had been grieving for a long time. When she started dying we'll never know. Since the cancer had spread to her lymph nodes four years after we had married, the cancer might have been present all the years of our fifteen-year marriage. I'm not sure when I began grieving her loss, but it was years before she died. Now I was grieving in a new way: mourning layered over grief. I needed to build a new life. Laurene had been right, I didn't want to be alone. I was happy going through life with a partner who knew what to do and where to go without getting lost.

Maybe I'll get married again. Someday, maybe.

I wanted to go somewhere. *I didn't know where "where" was.* I didn't want to go somewhere to get away. I wanted to find a place where I could be happy again. I recalled the happy night when I had proposed to Laurene. She wore a neck scarf and a navy blue suit. Her hair fell down to her shoulders. Her almond-shaped blue eyes sparkled in candlelight. We sat at a table for two covered with a white tablecloth. I opened a black velvet case, took out the blue sapphire ring bordered with diamonds, and placed it on her finger. She accepted. She said she loved me, because I listened and understood her better than anyone she had ever known. She said she loved the ring, because Princess Diana had worn a sapphire engagement ring. I had brought a camera to dinner, because I knew Laurene would want to take pictures.

I heard your wife died. Yes, she's dead. Sorry.

LESSON NINETEEN

**Grief involves thoughts and feelings about loss.
Mourning is the process of picking up the pieces.**

20.

I was about to take in anything
That the unveiled valley below,
Damp with tears of despair, was about to show
  me.

Dante's Inferno, Canto XX

I heaped up the bold prints and bright colors of Laurene's wardrobe, and placed them in the back of the Suburban. I drove to a consignment store on Shepherd Avenue. The store owner gave me a cold greeting, and almost refused to look at the clothes. She said she had a full inventory of seasonal clothes, and didn't need any more. Reluctantly, she walked out to the car. When I showed her the clothes, she changed her mind. She took all of them.

"I just wanted to get them out of the house. My wife died."

"You aren't the first man to lose a wife, and you won't be the last," she said.

Most people regard self pity as an undesirable feeling. It is a difficult emotion to accept. I had seldom experienced self pity before Laurene died, but every time I thought that the house had finally been cleared, other things continued to pop up that reminded me to feel sorry for myself. Her voice on the answering machine:

hello, this is Laurene.
you have reached the Evans residence.
we are away right now.
please leave a message.

Even now when I hear a central Texas accent, I'm reminded of the soft intonations of her voice. Even though Laurene had lived in the North for most of her adult life, she had never lost her accent. During the years I lived in Texas, I kept my Ohio accent, but I tried to pronounce Laurene's name the way she preferred. Most of the time, I called her *Lor-ene,* but her parents and childhood friends called her *Law-rene.* I wrote a haiku in my journal:

you die in the fall
your voice greeting still on
hear me say I love you.

Other than the woman in the consignment store, most people were more patient, kind, and treated me with natural goodness. But for months, I could not help but begin every new conversation with something that sounded like "Hello, I'm Randy. I lost my wife."

"I'm sorry for your loss," people would say. Even these well-meaning responses were unsatisfying to me. Their words sounded like a shallow and disconnected reflex. Perhaps the impolite comment by the woman at the consignment store was more honest and direct. To paraphrase Raymond Carver, *"How do we talk when we talk about loss?"*

In addition to the instrumental support she had given me in our marriage, Laurene had also been a base for my emotional support in the face of setbacks and disappointments. Faith in God might have helped, but I was angry with God. God served my need for an easy target. How could I get angry with Laurene? How could I get angry with cancer? God had let us down. How could a God let Laurene die? I wanted to believe that she was near and still alive in whatever Heaven happened to be. After all, I thought, *how could a good God create humans with eternal hope to disappoint us with death? It would be like building a car that could run forever, only to order it scrapped after a 100,000 miles.*

I revisited my faith once more. Faith had always been my last resort, a remote and barely accessible place that I would visit, only after my own pursuits had failed. *Where had my first confidence in the existence of God come from? Why had I been unable to sustain my faith?* On the way home from the consignment shop, I stopped the car at a park, and found a bench away from the noisy rush of traffic. I sat down and reflected. As a young boy in Akron, Ohio, I had felt transcendence standing on a high hill at the Hale Homestead during a weekend Scout camp out. The beauty of the fall color filled me with light and color. Still a child, I experienced a letting in rather than a looking out. I wasn't aware of the presence of God, but I felt something beyond my known world at the time—a mysterious, reassuring presence.

As an adult, my company had sent me to a personal growth lab in Bethel, Maine. One day, our facilitator led us on a shamanic journey to find our power animal. To the hypnotic beat of drums, we tried to connect with our power animals for two days. After getting over the fact that I thought the whole exercise was ridiculous, I let myself go through a dark tunnel into a different state of consciousness. I landed in a beaver lodge to find a disgruntled beaver who told me that he was in no way my power animal, and he shooed me away. This first attempt failed, but the vivid awareness of the experience impressed me.

On the second day, I shot out of everyday consciousness onto a fast-moving stream sparkling with sunlight. The heightened awareness of the day before returned. Lush green trees with overhanging branches lined the water's edge. Water sprayed on my face. I could see and smell water mist hanging over the waterline of the stream like a veil. Rough pebbles pressed against the bottoms of my feet. I had to brace my body to hold fast against the current. Suddenly on my left, a coyote appeared with sharp-pointed features, three feet on a large boulder and one foot raised in the air.

"Are you my power animal?" I said.

"Yes, I am your power animal."

The coyote turned towards me, and then turned to face downstream. I could see his long bushy tail. He pushed off from his right rear leg while his other legs moved forward in the air. He leapt into the stream.

I felt wild and free. I let my body splash into the stream and I swam alongside the coyote. The stream transported us fast and without effort. The rapid movement thrilled me. We drifted in tandem downstream on top of the water. After a long ride, we emerged to rest on a large rock. We both dripped stream water. The coyote's coat sparkled like stars in sunlight. "What's your name?" I said.

"GLISTEN," he said. *"MY NAME IS GLISTEN."*

"WHAT?"

"GLISTEN."

The coyote leaped into the woods, and I returned to waking consciousness.

The next day, I sat alone in our community room, puzzled by the power of what had happened. When I had given up trying to figure it out, insight arrived like the gift of a beautiful sunrise:

GLISTENS...GOD...LISTENS...GOD LISTENS.

A coyote named Glisten was a word contraction, sent to me by a God who loved me and understood me. He knew how my mind worked, because he made it. He had sent me a word selected for my own ears. God knew that I played with words like children played with toys. God knew that I would decipher the message. At the moment of insight, I felt the certain presence of God.

GOD LISTENS! God was on the other side of prayer after all. God would guide me through the rest of my life, and help me overcome my fears—fear of loss, fear of getting lost, fear of death, fear of going to hell, fear of rejection, fear of failure, fear of abandonment. I felt no need to prove what happened, or to discuss the experience with others. It was unemotional. The clouds didn't open up. No thunder clapped. It felt more like God had sent me an email with a yellow smiley-faced emoticon (hope not).

Now I needed to rekindle that faith, and at the same time, reach out to others in new ways. I could no longer depend on Laurene. I could no longer live in my thought bubble. I needed to remember all the family birthdays. I needed to learn how to make small talk about the news and sports. I had to attract new friends. I needed to find more people to love, and to learn how to receive love. I had always hidden behind my job—too busy to stay in touch, too busy to be informed, too busy to be intimate.

The week after the memorial service, everyone had left town. I wanted to leave town, too. It was hunting season in Texas, so I decided to drive from Houston to Brownwood to relax. Since there were no structures other than an old tool shed on the family farm, I took my tent along and set it up near the back of the property by an old stone fence line that had preceded the invention of barbed wire. There was a view of the tank Neil had bulldozed in the 1970s, and the hillside was shaded by mesquite trees.

The morning after I set up camp, I walked in darkness towards the middle of the farm, removed a piece of sheet metal that served as the tool shed door, and sat on a rusty folding chair inside to watch the sun rise. I had Neil's rifle with me, but I wasn't in the mood to hunt. While sitting there, an enormous blue eye appeared on the other side of the cutout window to my left.

A large brown paint horse stood outside the tool shed with a patch of white on its head. The horse looked at me. As I stepped out of the blind, the horse trotted towards the tank. Down by the water, another paint horse lowered its head to drink, then joined our procession around the fence line. We scared up some deer and a red fox, and in a swampy area, a snake spooked one of the horses. Rabbits jumped everywhere. I sighted a roadrunner in the brush. I passed the rotten hull of Neil's rowboat, a rusted overturned wheelbarrow, and piles of old brush. I rummaged around the ruins of a wind-scattered hunting blind. I uncovered the skeleton of a horny toad which looked like a small dinosaur, an empty metal ammo box, and two small arrowheads.

The way the blue-eyed horse fixed its bright eyes on me, I wanted to believe that the horse had been sent as a gift from Laurene. The horse raised its upper lip to show its teeth in a ghost of a smile. I knew nothing about horses, and certainly did not know whether horses smiled or not. Maybe that's how they smell. The horses let me pat them on their necks. They both looked healthy, like they had been fed and cared for by someone. I called the Brown County sheriff's office. No one had reported missing horses. I decided to name the smiling one "Blue."

"If you find an unclaimed animal on your property, you own it after 48 hours," the sheriff said.

So I now owned two horses. I visited my neighbor across the road, a dentist and goat farmer. He told me that people often placed animals on vacant property when they could no longer afford to feed them. He offered to throw alfalfa bales over the fence until I could decide what to do with the horses. He used the opportunity of our meeting to tell me that I needed a new fence.

"When you have fence down, you don't know what sorry maverick's gonna show up. All kinds of exotics get loose and roam around—aoudad and mouflon sheep, axis and fallow deer, blackbuck antelopes, not to mention rabid dogs, fox, coyote, wild pig—and an occasional mountain lion or even a panther roaming up from Old Mexico. A good fence won't keep all the varmints out, but without one you might as well hang a big welcome sign by the road. I know a good fence builder in town. Here's his number. Let me know if you decide to use him, because I can help you. He cheats on pricing, so you have figure out what you're willing to pay in advance. He measures off the fence line riding an old mule, which leaves a lot of room for his estimates."

A few months later, I moved both horses to a horse farm near town. I returned a few times to check on them, and the owner would take me riding. She insisted that I ride her daughter's horse, because my two horses were unbroken. She taught me how mount and dismount, and how to lean in the saddle going up and down hills. I enjoyed riding through the rolling countryside from atop a horse. At the end of the rides, I would visit Blue in a corral. She had bites all over her flank, a victim of a more dominant horse who wanted to assert the pecking order of the herd, the owner said. Blue hadn't figured out how to be subservient. She was used to freedom.

I kept going back to Brownwood over the next three months. Each time, I stopped at the cemetery to visit Laura Schmitt's grave. One late afternoon, a middle-aged woman stood in the cemetery holding a mix of wild flowers in her shaking hands. The haphazard assortment looked hand-picked. The woman stood over a plot piled high with fresh dirt while she cried. We stood in the shade of the huge oak tree, and avoided eye contact.

We're both under the long curve of human suffering, the never-ending process of grieving that tails out towards infinity, or at least in our case, to the end of our lives. We stood under the shadow of the oak tree, and grieved separately in our own way.

The woman and I nodded to each other, and we returned to our cars. I could have stopped to talk with her. She might have been a relative of someone who had lived in Jordan Springs before the town had disappeared. Maybe she had known Neil or Stella, not unlikely in a small town. Maybe we could have engaged in small talk, or more importantly, shared our fresh grief. Had she been with us, Laurene would have talked to this woman. I did not.

A Husband's Passage Through Cancerland

One cold morning in 1969, I was sitting in a subway clacking along from 34th Street to 116th on my way to class at Columbia. I sat shoulder to shoulder with a black woman, about my age. Our bodies leaned in to each other from time to time as we sat on the bench seat for over thirty minutes. The subway lurched from one local stop to the next on its way uptown. Reflected in the opposite windows, I could see our four eyeballs bounce sideways at each stop to see the numbers of the stops displayed on the subway tiles, the nines and sixes of 96th Street, and so on. Her body warmed me. What if I had talked with that woman, maybe about the weather or the news, or what if our conversation had resulted in an intimate exchange, or an insight that might have changed our lives in a small or big way? How many times in my life had I missed opportunities for love and joy by failing to engage with others in moments like these?

I need to work on relationships. I must lower the barriers that distance me from others. I need to develop the capacity to connect with others on my own. I had let Laurene be the part of me that reached out to other people.

LESSON TWENTY

As people disappear from your life, you become aware of the part of them that was, and still is, a part of you.

21.

He strode the length of the bridge
To the bank of the sixth crevice; at that point,
He needed to look like he knew what he was doing.
Could I have safely come this far
In spite of the countless obstacles
Unless I'd been guided by divine will and a promise of success?
Let us through. Heaven wants me
To show someone this soul-crushing way.

Dante's Inferno, Canto XXI

Jeremy and Laura drove down to Brownwood from Colorado Springs the week before Christmas. Jeremy and I hunted rabbits, and we spent a full day clearing an area to build a wooden platform for my tent. The platform consisted of eight 4X8 sheets of plywood nailed to a 2x4 frame. We placed the tent on the platform, and slept together in our new campsite.

The next day, Billy Connaway rolled up the dirt road in his golf cart while we were fixing breakfast over an open fire. When he took off his dirty white cowboy hat, a stark red tan line ran across his forehead. He didn't say hello or introduce himself. Of course, I had met him a few months before when I had busted the chain on his gate.

"Whad'ya build that for?" he said.

"I wanted to keep my tent off the ground...to get away from the jiggers and ticks...the fire ants, and spiders." I felt like I had done something wrong. "And to keep the snakes away," I added by way of further justification.

"Son, you're buildin' yourself one of the finest snake hotels in the entire county. All the snakes 'round here will be telling their friends and relations to come on in under this floor and get out of the sun. They'll be havin' parties on Saturday nights."

"I haven't seen any snakes around here," I said. Laura's eyes expanded, and she started to look around for snakes. I shifted my feet nervously.

"We have lots of snakes around here. They crawl around by the tanks, unless of course they can find something more attractive like underneath this here deck. When I was a boy, we swam in them tanks all the time."

"What about the snakes?" I said. "You swam with snakes?"

"Always had enough room for everyone in them tanks. The thing you got to know about snake...snakes don't take kindly to bein' stomped on. Cattle kill snakes all the time. They don't mean to...it's a natural accident. What you have to do is take a heavy stick when you walk, and keep knockin' the ground with it. A snake will think cattle. Snakes don't want trouble. They jest don' want to be crawling around and get kicked in the head or squashed."

"I'll remember that." Laura began to look for a stick.

"That's not why I came over. My ticker's broke down, and I'm goin' to die soon. I knew Neil and Stella all my life. Stella's my cousin. I knew their girl, too...Laurene. She always wore a dress, because her grandfather didn't want to see girls in shorts. She kept up with the boys, and Stella would scold her, because she always had mud on her dress. We boys would take her down to the tank in an old wagon, and we'd all splash around. Laurene would say, 'Momma's going to be mad when she sees my dress.' She wasn't at all afraid of snakes or much of anything else as I remember. I knew she'd be someone even when we were children. She wasn't the kind that stands around holdin' a floor down. Well, anyway, no one wants my land after I die, so you might consider buyin' it. The two properties used to be together a long time ago——before barbed wire. One stone wall 'round the whole place. My Daddy sold a piece to Neil so he could reach the road by car. Momma didn't want to sell the land, but Daddy always liked Neil."

"Thanks," I said. "Thanks, for thinking of me. I'll let you know." He turned the golf cart around. Jeremy and I joined Laura's search for walking sticks. Billy had traveled about fifty yards back down the fence line in the direction of the road, before he turned around and headed back to us. He pulled up to the snake hotel.

"I s'pose you know you need a new fence," he said. "There's a good fence man in town, but let me handle him for you. He builds the best fence in the county, but he's known to overcharge, especially since he measures the fence line while he rides on a mule. Next time you come, look me up and I'll show you where Neil and his mother's house used to be, and I'll show you an old map of the property. There's an Indian burial mound in the back. Used to be a village here 'til the Rangers ran 'em out. And one more thing, did you know Camp Bowie used this land for an artillery range during WWII? I wouldn't worry much about snakes, but an unexploded shell could ruin your whole day. If you find one and it doesn't blow up on you, be sure to call the Army."

He trailed off in his golf cart again, then he hesitated, and placed his head against the steering wheel as if he was thinking about one more thing to tell us. What more stories about this land resided in his mind? His cart rumbled its way to the road, and his big white hat disappeared. He died three weeks later along with many more untold stories. A few months later, I bought his property, and hired the mule man to build a six-strand fence. The following year, I received a letter from the US Army. They had scheduled the land for inspection each year for forty years, but hadn't gotten around to it because of budget restrictions. If they ever did, they wanted my permission to come on the property. I have never heard from them again. Over the years, I've unearthed dozens of arrowheads, forged nails, old coins, the flattened skeleton of a horned lizard, but no artillery shells.

Jennifer, Nathan, and Meredith joined us in Houston for Christmas. Jeremy made a stew from our rabbits on Christmas Eve. We opened a few presents, attended a candle lighting service at church, and returned home to watch movies. On Christmas morning, we fixed breakfast together, and instead of my usual rubbery scrambled eggs, we placed soft and delicious Eggs Benedict on the table. The next day, we drove to downtown Houston to see "A Christmas Carol," and to celebrate Jennifer and Nathan's first wedding anniversary. We didn't need to discuss how and what we did for Christmas, because there was an unspoken agreement that we would follow Laurene's holiday routines. I began to dread the departures.

"Dad, you're coming back to Colorado with me," Laura said. Laura surprised me with such a bold instruction. She had decided to take care of me, to bring me to her home. At first I wanted to resist, but I had no reason to stay in a house that no longer felt like home. I thought, *why not? The memorial service is over. Everyone's left. The days between Christmas and New Years are empty I have nothing but time.* I felt relieved, almost giddy, about leaving town without a purpose other than to be with people I loved, like I had been relieved of active duty.

So Jeremy and Laura drove me from Houston to Colorado Springs. I slept in the backseat for the better part of the sixteen-hour drive. I hadn't realized how exhausted I was—out cold after one yawn. When we arrived at their bungalow in the historic district, Laura made a bed for me on the living room sofa. Jeremy and Laura had recently moved into their first house. The 100-year-old bungalow sat about eight blocks from the Colorado College campus and downtown Colorado Springs. Pike's Peak back dropped their yard. I felt happy to be with two people who loved me.

For two or three hours every morning for the next week, I walked the tree-shaded streets of Colorado Springs. I memorized the street grid. I found the bayou, the parks, the coffee shops, the book stores, the fountains, the park benches, and the street people. For me, walking became a healing ritual. I had always been a runner, but it was slow walking that helped heal me. I breathed in the mountain air, and exhaled my grief. I felt less overwhelmed, less lonely. On my walks, I thought about what to do next. I intended to visit the rest of the children—Nathan and Jennifer in Grand Rapids, Amy in Cleveland, and Meredith in Nashville. Meredith would be graduating from Vanderbilt in May.

Along my daily walking route, I passed a yoga and massage studio. One day I scheduled a massage. After a short interview, the therapist took me into a small room and told me to undress and lay face down under a sheet. The room was dark without lamps, or candles, or windows—the blackest dark one could imagine. The pressure of the therapist's hands on my skin and muscles emptied my head. She startled me when she asked me to turn over face up. I may have fallen asleep.

While the therapist sat on a stool behind me and began massaging my scalp, I opened my eyes and stared into the black space. Laurene appeared. She walked towards me. Dressed in white, a white light surrounded her. Her face formed a cheerful, almost triumphant, smile. She stood so near. She said nothing, but she looked at me in the familiar had exchange glances through the course of our relationship, with a bemused brightness in our eyes; the same looks we had exchanged when we first saw each other after her mastectomy so many years before, or after returning from one of our long business trips. Even though she was washed in light, she looked like herself. I think Laurene wanted me to know that she was still hanging around, a simple text message from the great beyond.

I'm not going to try to explain why or how this happened, but rather to report that it happened in the way I explained—not as a meeting, or a revelation, or a dream, but more as a fact, a crystal clear awareness of my dead wife's presence, like the awareness of God that I had experienced in Maine. I had the evidence of my experience, and that was all I needed. Laurene appeared calm and peaceful. She looked healthy and free of pain.

She was not what I imagined as an angel, but simply the figure of the imperfect woman who had loved me, and argued and pushed me around to get her way. I don't think she wanted me to idealize her in death any more than she had refused to let me idealize her in life. A few months before she died, we had visited her favorite aunt in Cleveland, Texas. At the memorial service, Aunt Lucille told me what Laurene had said to her during the visit: "Randy spoils me just like my Daddy spoiled me."

Maybe she had broken some heaven rule by coming back to see me?

I walked back to have dinner with Jeremy and Laura. The sun was still shining, and there was a light breeze. My heart was lighter. It made me happy to experience a world after this world in so concrete a way, and to know that our relationship with loved ones who have passed needn't end at a locked door, to know that time's line doesn't travel a one-way street. And the mystery of it all reassured me. Just like untold stories that Billy Connaway had carried to the grave, and the buried artifacts under the farm in Brownwood, the universe had its own secrets.

I'm ready to move on. Rather than dwelling on memories, and mourning the life we had that is no more, Laurene is still with me. There is no reason to be unhappy for the small span of time I have yet to live.

I traveled on to Grand Rapids, and spent a few days with Jennifer and Nathan. They were kind to me. I felt take care of in the same way that Laura and Jeremy had nurtured me in Colorado.

I thought I had turned the corner until we went to see *Shadowlands* at the cinema in Grand Rapids. We didn't know that the movie was about a man who had lost his wife to cancer—the love relationship between CS Lewis (played by Anthony Hopkins) and American Poet Joy Davidman (played by Debra Winger), and her tragic death from cancer. Once we got out to the car, I broke down and sobbed. Nathan

Out of the Inferno

placed his hand on my arm, and asked if there was anything he could do.

A Husband's Passage Through Cancerland

LESSON TWENTY-ONE

Grief returns in circles and spheres, in unexpected ways, and opens what you thought had been a locked door.

22.

'Uh-oh! That one's showing his teeth!
I'd love to keep chatting but I'm afraid
He's getting ready to carve his initials in my
*   neck.'*

Dante's Inferno, Canto XXII

When Nathan touched my arm and offered his assistance, I felt comforted. My new sons-in-laws had been very supportive since Laurene's passing. On the plane to Nashville, I thought about how few male friends I had in my life, and what I had missed.

My brother was my first and only life-long friend. Eighteen months younger, Dave and I had played together every day through our school years. I didn't need to seek out other playmates so much, because we had each other. My parents called Dave, "Little Me Too," because what ever I wanted he wanted. We played baseball, basketball, backyard football, and ping pong together. Attended summer camp together. We got in trouble together, sneaking out of our bed at night to chase lightning bugs on the lawn or look in the neighbor's windows.

Then I met George in grade school, the grandson of a Serbian shepherd, and we became best friends though junior high. We shared our expanding knowledge about everything from sex to Santa Claus. We shared dirty jokes, and faked farts with our arm pits. He played the tenor sax and I played the clarinet. His grandfather took us to "professional" wrestling matches at the Akron Arena on Saturday nights. We camped out in his backyard under the watchful eye of his grandfather. We trolled the neighborhood visiting our favorite girl friends. We listened to 45 records, traded comic books, baseball cards, and tried to dance.

Our fathers enrolled us in a body building class, because we were both pudgy. Every Saturday, we took an Akron City bus down Market Street. We dragged Warner, our skinny friend, along for the ride. The trolleybus screeched on overhead electric wires stopping a dozen times on the way to the Y. On one of the stops, we exited the bus to buy a bag of donuts at the Krispy Kreme Donut Factory. Once we arrived at Central YMCA, we found an empty wrestling room, and each downed three donuts during the bodybuilding class. We liked to swim, so from eleven to twelve we joined the other naked swimmers in the pool to finish in time for lunch at a local diner across the street from the Y. Our fathers kept looking for muscle definition, but our muscles stayed safely cushioned behind layers of fat during elementary school until we leaned down as teenagers.

One day, Dad found Dave and me behind the garage, poking each other in the privates with the knob end of a baseball bat. He went berserk. We were surprised by the intensity of his reaction. We got the very clear message that touching another boy in any way was wrong. I later learned the meaning of homophobia. I don't think Dad forgot the incident, because in later years, he shared a story of how a sailor had goosed him on his destroyer in the middle of the Pacific in WWII, and how he had dragged the sailor down three flights of metal stairs. Shortly before Dad died, he told me how during the Depression, relatives stayed at his house over weekends. Since my grandfather was a grocer, everyone came over for meals. Dad said that one of his uncles had slept in his bed. He said that his uncle was an evil man. I had never heard him call anyone evil before. That's all he said.

So I grew up with a problem. I didn't get close to boys or later in life, other men, not in any worthwhile way. I played football and ran track, participated in other school activities, but never discussed problems, admitted fears, shared concerns, or heaven forbid, mentioned failures with men; since women were a mystery to me, I had no where to go for emotional support. On the other hand, Dad and the other men in my life, schooled me to compete. Dad told me to distinguish myself in small ways (be clean and dress well, work harder than the next guy), and in big ways (get better grades, stay in better shape, arrive at work early and stay late, volunteer for special assignments, and do a quality job). He told me never to fumble for something in my pockets, because people would regard me as disorganized. Keep your wallet in your back left pocket, have a clean handkerchief in your back right pocket, keep change in your right front pocket, and a pocket knife in your front left pocket. Keep your pencils sharp, and don't buy leaky pens. Be wary of strangers. "Fool me once shame on you, fool me twice, shame on me" were his words to live by.

While my mother encouraged friendships with both girls and boys, she couldn't overcome the defenses set up by my father, and the fathers of the other boys. You could see them all cheering us on during baseball practice, and giving the refs a rough time for bad calls. They bragged about us. They criticized us. They hardened us. When we injured ourselves, the mantra that came from the stands: *"LAUGH IT OFF! LAUGH IT OFF.!"*

Crying was the worst thing you could do. One day, a school friend fell off an eight-foot stone wall that bordered our school yard. He fell on his back and lost his wind. He cried. All of us boys stood there and looked at him, and then walked away. He had broken the cardinal rule that had glowed like a neon sign over my childhood: *BIG BOYS DON'T CRY.* So I learned to keep feelings to myself, and to never show weakness, especially to other boys who could be future competitors. One day, I pitched out the class bully in a baseball game. He came after me with his bat. Our coach let him approach the pitcher's mound. He wanted to see me defend myself. I kicked the kid in the balls, and this pleased the coach. With a mock smile on his face, he said, *"ARE YOU BOYS FIGHTING?"*

So the two life lessons for boys growing up in the fifties*: DON'T BE GAY AND DON'T BE A PUSHOVER.* Others boys, and later, other men, served as your competitors. You needed to assert yourself, and learn how to win, and keep winning—to get to the top and stay on the top. This is why men of my generation don't have friends. This is why women unfairly carry the overwhelming burden of a man's needs for emotional support and companionship. Male-to-male friendships are too rare.

When I started dating, I found out what I had been missing. Girls not only smelled better than boys, but they were great listeners, and fun to be around. They could take you into their basements and teach you how to dance and how to French kiss—until their mothers showed up carrying a load of laundry and threatening looks. Who needed boys for anything other than games? Boys were for competitive games and sports. Intimacy, warmth, and affection were reserved for girls, and if you were lucky, an occasional game of spin the bottle.

I liked girls so much that I idealized them. I placed my first wife on a pedestal so high that I didn't really know her. She was the first girl I had dated seriously. We attended college together. We dated seven years before we married after my first year in graduate school at Columbia. I heaped the weight of my emotional and social needs on her until after fifteen years, the weight destroyed our marriage.

As I traveled with my job and worked long hours, my goal was to distinguish myself, and climb the corporate ladder on schedule. Buy a house and own a car. Buy a bigger house and own a bigger car. Have one child, and then another. Learn to play golf, and join a country club. Stay fit enough to be a threat, hold my liquor, and puff on a cigar once in awhile to be one of the boys.

I did not display pictures of my wife and children in my office. Exposing affection for your family showed a lack of focus on the job, a reason to get passed over for a promotion. The advantage of marriage in the corporate world had less to do with the support of a loving family, than with the appearance of stability: a mortgage meant you had to earn money to make payments, kids in school meant you had to save for college—and all of this translated to the need for job security, the need to keep your job under any circumstances, even if you had to do things that weren't always right. The need for money and job security reduced the likelihood that you would ask unwanted questions or otherwise become a troublemaker. You knew you had made it when the higher ups called you a straight arrow.

But when Nathan touched my arm, I felt his expression of warmth as something new and welcome. No longer a taboo. The right touch at the right time, and his offer to help, altered my expectations about the benefits of male friendships. But I still had more confidence in the support of a woman.

***

Before I left Grand Rapids, I dropped down to Kalamazoo for breakfast with Denise, a woman that I had worked with at Haworth beginning in the 1980s. Denise had left Haworth to head the human resources department of a successful medical equipment manufacturer. A mutual friend informed me that Denise was now with Pfizer and that I should look her up while I was in Michigan. I called Denise, and we met for breakfast by the airport where she had a meeting scheduled with the Pfizer Flight Department. She had been a single mother for fifteen years after marrying at age nineteen. Dana, her daughter, was in college. I asked her if 7:30 AM was too early. She reminded me of my Monday morning 7:00 AM staff meetings when she had to get Dana to a sitter before school.

We enjoyed breakfast. Even though we had worked together for six years, Denise seemed like someone new. I had never noticed her expressiveness. She displayed so many different facial expressions as she talked. You could sell tickets to see her repertoire of faces. She looked attractive, professional, and self confident. She had moved up since leaving Haworth. She had been underweight at Haworth, and now she looked healthy and fit. She drove a big new car, and owned a beautiful house. She co-owned an airplane with her father, a Piper Arrow, and had joined a flying club. She worked out with a personal trainer. She was taking kayaking lessons. She had recently traveled to Italy with her sisters. I have never been especially perceptive about picking up details, but while she talked, I noticed her dark brown hair and big expressive eyes. To my later dismay, I didn't pick up the color of her eyes, a nearly fatal mistake.

I wasn't surprised when Denise told me that there had been actors in her family, and that she had studied drama in college. She entertained me, and made me laugh. She cheered me up. She talked about her job, her daughter, her sisters, her parents, and her cat and dog. When she told me she was sorry to hear that Laurene died, I didn't feel like she said so to be polite. She talked straight. I let her words sink in without dismissing her good intentions. She said that Debby, her sister, had recently been diagnosed with glioblastoma, an aggressive brain cancer. Her face softened as she spoke. I could tell that she loved her family.

I looked for a wink of encouragement, but found no signs that she wanted to see me again. She seemed happy to see me, but nothing more. Maybe she had a boyfriend? Maybe she didn't like me? Maybe I had somehow offended her in the past? Maybe she was plain busy, and had no time for old acquaintances? We ended breakfast abruptly, because she had to leave for her meeting. I felt a tinge of jealousy about how engaged she was in her job. She still lived the life I had once led—active, focused, in demand by others. I thought I would give her a call after I returned to Houston. I liked her.

I visited Amy in Chagrin Falls, Ohio next. We spent some time shopping and having lunch in the place I had lived for three years between my first and second marriages. I knew every building—each restaurant, retail shop, church, grocery store, and the masonic lodge. My oldest daughter and I enjoyed reminiscing about her childhood in the area, and our Indian Princess campouts along the Mohican River when all four girls had camped with me in a single tent on a stormy weekend, when Amy had spilled an entire liter of Coke inside the tent.

After Amy and I said good-bye, I walked around the town for an hour as I had done in Colorado Springs. Walking in the midst of people running errands, standing in the middle of things that happen every day, comforted me. I remembered taking the girls on a roller coaster at the fair beside the river, and the cotton candy sticking to our fingers in the summer heat. This was the last place I had been single—where I had ended a marriage and started a new one. I stopped at the bridge to watch the Chagrin River flow over the falls with its load of fallen limbs and other debris. White plastic bags, half-empty beer cans, bits of garbage, and yard waste dotted the fast flowing water. A discarded tire pushed by leaving a small wake. No one would want to photograph a river floating with trash, but I thought all taking all this in represented real life, which is never picture perfect.

Maybe it's not best to take in everything at once (in the depths of the Inferno, Virgil had placed his hands protectively over Dante's eyes), but eventually you have to take everything in. Then you see the whole of life—the good and bad, the ripe and rotten, the good looking and the unattractive. Even if you tried to hide the unsightly stuff, it would not be possible. Even though the river carried trash, the air above the river smelled fresh and new. I wanted back into the whole dirty mess of living again. Even though the sky was a leaden gray, I felt like I might be heading towards sunshine.

Maybe Denise would be my sunshine?

LESSON TWENTY-TWO

The prescription for isolation is contact.

23.

From the rock rim, he slid on his back
Down the incline that forms the dividing wall
That borders the sixth pocket.
Water never rushed so fast...

Dante's Inferno, Canto XXIII

When I arrived in Nashville to visit Meredith, she had nearly finished her college education. Her sisters and I had been worried about her, because she hadn't talked much about losing her mother. I took her girlfriends out for a hilarious lunch where I shared funny stories of Meredith's childhood, and revealed her family nickname, "Mer Bear." When we were alone, I asked how she was doing.

"I'm okay. I know Mom's in heaven, and I know she still loves me."

Meredith was doing fine. Her matter-of-fact response disarmed me. The simplicity of her faith had to be the real answer to the question of grief. She spoke of her mother in the present tense. She was not trying to get closure about or to get over her mother's death. Grieving had become a natural part of her life, a form of loving her mother in a different way. You can learn much from your children.

And she had lots of friends.

I flew back to Houston. I kept thinking about the bright radiance of Denise's ever-changing face. I would have to give her a call.

I had always thought that I would be strong enough to be alone, but loneliness leaked in. One by one the light bulbs in my house popped out. The lights where Laurene and I had spent the most time blacked out first. I didn't change them. I preferred sitting in the dark without the decorative reminders of my past life. One night, the pool emptied for no known cause. A few days later, a section of brick fell off the house. My old life was falling apart around me.

I kept thinking about Denise. I wanted to call her on an upbeat day, when I would sound confident and good humored over the phone. I worried that she might politely dismiss me, and that would be the end. I tried to distract myself with all the stuff sitting inside and outside the house, all the remnants of the past fifteen years and before: the trampoline that I bought Meredith as a consolation for her mother's absences in Houston, old bicycles, a Sunfish sailboat, boxes of mementoes, cookbooks and recipes, Royal Doulton figurines, a silver tea service, a chocolate fountain. I even found the engraved napkins from Laurene's wedding to John.

I started going through the house from top to bottom. I tagged items: "KEEP," "DONATE," "TRASH," "NOT SURE." In the attic, I found the suitcases filled with the girls' clothes that they had protected from my poor laundering during Laurene's out-of-town treatments. I opened the attic window and threw empty corrugated computer and electronics boxes into the side yard for disposal. I found a high chair, a crib, and a doll cradle made by Dad for the girls. In a corner against the rafters, cross country skis stood, equipment from our early years in Michigan. Would I ever move back North? I decided to keep them. In our bedroom closet, I found more cash hidden in the back of a dresser drawer.

I signed up for a Feldenkrais body movement class at the Jung Center in the Museum District. The exercises relaxed me, but when I looked around me, I observed a sea of bright-colored exercise clothes worn by young mothers. I felt alone and conspicuous. I bought a series of tickets to the Houston Symphony. I revisited the museums, and sat through movies. I went out on a few dates with various women that I had run across in one way or another, but no one inspired me like Denise had. My feeble attempts at playing the field left me more alone and dissatisfied.

I visited an online dating site, but scrolling through the profiles made me feel depressed and voyeuristic. I didn't know how to answer the questions:

What do I do for fun? (JOG). What job? (NO JOB). My religion? (MOSTLY METHODIST), Favorite hot spots? (HOT TUB). Favorite things? (PITCHING WEDGE), Last read? (*YOUR GUIDE TO PLANNING MEANINGFUL FUNERALS*), Age range of women I am seeking? (MY AGE PLUS 5 OR MINUS 15), Marital status? (SINGLE? WIDOWED? WIDOWERED?), Kids? (FOUR DAUGHTERS WHO MAY HATE YOU), Body type? (I CAN SEE MY FEET), Daily diet? (PALEO DIET SANS FRUITS, VEGETABLES, NUTS, AND SEEDS), Body art? (APPENDECTOMY SCAR AND A MOLE THAT LOOKS LIKE THE VIRGIN MARY), Astrological sign? (SCORPIO I THINK), Pets? (AN OLD DIABETIC CAT), Smoke? (CIGARS OUTDOORS), Dance? (*YMCA* AT WEDDINGS).

Who would want me? And even worse, if someone wanted me, what kind of person would they be? I kept thinking about Denise. I felt an uncomplicated affection for her. I didn't idealize her. Thinking about her simply made me feel cheerful inside, like a crisp middle C struck on a piano. Already knowing most of the answers to the online dating questions, would she be interested in me in a new way? Would she make me dance?

I waited a few weeks to call her back. I thought about how we might fit as a couple. *Boring and serious,* that's what she probably thought about me. Once at Haworth, we had played a guessing game about our pasts, and Denise had disclosed that she had been a cheerleader in high school. The cheerleaders in my high school only dated the guys on the varsity sports teams. Excluded from the popular clique, I had felt like an outsider. I had been on the debate team, not of great interest to the cheerleaders. I had played the lead role in *Teahouse of the August Moon,* but Captain Fisby had not been invited to the cast party. Denise liked to dance and have fun. I preferred to sit quietly and read a book. I didn't think that I would have any more of a chance with Denise, than I had with the cheerleaders in high school.

At home in Houston, I jogged every morning before breakfast. I lunched with a few men in my neighborhood, and played some golf, a depressing sport unless you have a low handicap. A woman down the street invited me to play bridge (I didn't know how). A couple asked me out to dinner, but I felt awkward filling a table for three. I continued my training sessions at the fitness center. My young female trainer had arm muscles bigger than my thigh muscles. I didn't progress much more than when my Dad had sent me to body building classes in grade school, because the work outs made me crave jelly donuts or butter-toasted Everything Bagels with cream cheese.

I trained with the Literacy Volunteers of America, and began working with Latino boys on their English skills. I tutored statistics at the community college. These activities were fun, but not enough to occupy my time and energy. I took my pontoon boat out on Lake Conroe to catch crappie, white bass, and catfish. I bought a kayak and paddled on Lake Woodlands. I invited Laurene's doctor and his assistant out for a thank-you lunch at a fancy restaurant near the clinic. I bought some new clothes. I went to church and sobbed through the service. I joined a singles group at church without finding anyone of interest. I floated from one thing to another.

One day, I called Laurene's therapist to see about grief counseling. For some reason, the approach that he had taken with Laurene was not the approach he used with me. Rather than non-directive listening, he gave me more advice than I wanted to hear. I wanted to discuss new directions for my life, different sources of meaning and purpose, new and different relationships—drastic changes in all directions. He cautioned me against big changes. He urged me not to relocate or sell my house. He wanted me to avoid spending money without thinking things through. He thought returning to my business career might be a good idea. And more than anything else, he lectured me about dating. "You won't be ready to date for at least a year," he said, "and maybe not even then."

I had been running in place for over ten years. The last thing in the world that I wanted to do was nothing at all. The days of sitting in the waiting rooms were over. Over the next two years for better or worse, I ignored every one of his prescriptions.

The therapy session created a need for counseling. I had to talk with someone. I called Denise. Since our breakfast meeting at the airport, I had become more hopeful. False optimism had been a lifelong signature strength, but I could feel my heart racing as the phone rang. The bright sunlight outside my home office window slapped up against the house. My whole body squinted.

"Hello, this is Denise," she said in a professional voice.

"Hello, Denise. This is Randy."

"Hi..." *(no hint of interest)*

"How've you been?" *(my effort at small talk)*

"Good." *(one word responses are the kiss of death)*

"I enjoyed our breakfast the other week." *(so what?)*

"Me too." *(hint of interest?)*

"I'd like to see you again." *(too direct?)*

"I'm not your type." *(my worst fears confirmed)*

"What?" *(defer the inevitable)*

"I'm not your type." *(curtains)*

"I disagree." *(don't give up).*

"I'm an extrovert; you're an introvert. You want someone to have long intellectual conversations with—that's not me. Right now, I'm filling out my brackets for March Madness—do you want a woman who follows basketball? Do you know what a bracket is?" *(abandon all hope)*

"Of course, I know what a bracket is...although I've never filled one out—" *(last ditch effort)*

"—have you seen *Young Frankenstein*? *(what the hell? Is she giving me a test?)*

"That's a movie, right?" *(am I close?)*

"If you don't know Mel Brooks' humor, how could we have much in common?" *(Is he like Woody Allen?)*

"I've heard of Mel Brooks. Didn't he direct *Three Amigos?*" *(yes?)*

"No. John Landis."

"So your ideal man would sit around and talk about movies?" *(too defensive)*

"That would be good...so tell me what do you like about me?" *(a lifeline?)*

"You're sharp and fun and I love your blue eyes." *(that should wow her)*

*"My eyes are brown." **(OH NO!)***

"What's brown?" *(disbelief)*

"My eyes. Not even the doofuses I dated in high school got my eye color wrong." *(the curtain has dropped)*

"Oh." *(resignation)*

Oh, boy. What an idiot! All these weeks, and this is how you handled a simple phone call? She will never see me again. How could I get her eye color wrong? I worked with her for years, and never noticed her eye color? Laurene had blue eyes. My daughters had blue eyes. My first wife had blue eyes. There had never been a brown-eyed woman in my life. I might as well give up and hang up. She's eight years younger than me. Are we both Boomers? I don't hear dial tone. At least she hadn't hung up on me.

"I'd like to see you again, too," she said. "I'll be in Chicago two weeks from Friday on business. I'll meet you in the lobby of the W Hotel on Saturday morning at nine o'clock." *(Hallelujah! Hallelujah! Hallelujah!)*

"Okay," I said.

"Oh, I've got to go to a meeting." Denise hung up without saying good-bye. She never said good-bye on the telephone, and most of the time, she didn't say good-bye in person. She didn't like small talk.

I couldn't believe my good luck. In a matter-of-fact tone, Denise informed me that she had an upcoming business trip scheduled to Chicago. We could meet there on the weekend after she had finished with her meetings. I'd have to make my own lodging arrangements. I had no trouble booking a flight from Houston to Chicago after the telephone call ended. I registered at the Drake Hotel.

In the meantime, I called Denise a few times a week. Sometimes we talked for over an hour. She gave me entertaining accounts of her work at Pfizer, and of the people she worked with, describing each one in detail. She told me how she approached problems and decisions. Every call included an update on Dana, her daughter, and news about her parents, John and Audrey, and her sisters, Diane and Debby. Her father sounded like a man with a thousand retirement projects, from yard work to flying his airplane. Audrey busied herself with church work and a water aerobics group called the Water Lilies.

Denise asked me lots of questions about my desire to go back to school, about the farm in Brownwood, and about my family and friends. I enjoyed reporting my life to her. One evening after we had been talking for about twenty minutes, she asked me to do something for her. She wanted me to start calling her every day. I felt the same way. Even though we had been physically separate, each phone call closed the distance between us. Her voice was almost as expressive as her face.

"I can't wait to see your beautiful brown eyes in Chicago," I said one evening.

"Don't you ever forget the color of my eyes," she said.

***

We grabbed a taxi to the Museum of Science and Industry in Jackson Park. Growing up in Chicago's suburbs, Denise knew the sprawling museum like a well-trained docent, and could recount its history going back to the late eighteen hundreds. She said that she had been to the museum countless times on school field trips as a young girl. We spent a half day hitting her favorite places. We spent a long time viewing

Colleen Moore's Fairy Castle doll house. We looked in every miniature room. The rooms of the doll house represented the rooms of Denise's imaginary world: children's stories, animal fantasy tales, and Hollywood glamour.

Denise was enthusiastic and excited to share this vast world of exhibition halls. She talked about the exhibits as if she had created them—D-Day Normandy, Farm Technology, Ships Through the Ages, the U-505 Submarine, the Coal Mine, and the Baby Chick Hatchery. You could tell that she had planned our visit in advance as a way of opening a door to her world. Next to the doll house, her other other favorite exhibits, the 999 Empire Express steam locomotive, the WWII warplanes, and farm technology, represented Denise's love of flying, her interest in history, and her love of animals. The museum offered me an exterior map of her interior life.

For me, the walk through the museum with Denise proved to be a metaphor for what our future might be like. Even though Denise had a route in mind, she stopped to take advantage of special exhibits, or other newer exhibits that piqued her interest. She planned, but also improvised. She spoke clearly to me, and asked me what I thought about what we observed. In subtle ways, she laid out a way of being together that included fun, companionship, respect, and spontaneity. As the hours progressed, I felt less nervous about what she thought of me. I had the impression that she already had figured me out, and decided that I was an exception to her general view of men, which was not favorable.

I looked at her face, and thought, *there is nothing browner than her eyes.*

As we continued our walk through the vast exhibition halls, Denise talked about her family. Our travels through the museum included Denise's recounts of her youth living on the grounds of Elim Christian School in Palos Heights, a school for children and adults with special needs. Denise's father had been director of the school for his entire career beginning in 1950. The three girls had been surrounded by acres of playgrounds, stables, and classroom buildings. There were cats and dogs and ponies. Denise had cleaned out the horse stalls in the mornings before getting on the school bus. She knew how to fix broken machines. Her grandmother taught her how to cook in the school kitchen. She followed her father everywhere. He was a good teacher. He taught her how to fly. He loved her. Later he would repeat his favorite descriptor: "Denise is the one in our family who has her feet on the ground."

Denise had lived in one of the residential units, and worked at the school after graduating from college. She had worked with a wide range of physical and developmental disabilities—children with autism, hearing impairment, Tourette syndrome, and many with multiple disabilities. Hearing Denise's animated accounts of her childhood, I began to appreciate her abiding love of people. She could see behind physical and mental deformities, and the human flaws of people in general. Her tolerance for a wide range of human differences filled me with admiration and also with hope. I had always felt different from other people, and I was different from Denise—quiet, conservative, unexpressive, and eight years older. If she could love all kinds of people, maybe she could love me?

That evening, Denise took me out to dinner at The Italian Village, a Chicago landmark restaurant opened in 1927, where boys had taken her on high school dates. Maybe she chose this place as another way of connecting me to her past. The Village contained three restaurants under one roof. Denise chose the oldest of the three, a magical space decorated with wall murals depicting an Italian village and Lombardy Poplars against a gibbous moon and night sky. Tiny electric lights peeped from the windows of castles. Ornate flower boxes hung between Doric columns. Sparkling overhead lights hung from the ceiling on garish blue clouds. Denise listed all the celebrities who had dined at the restaurant: Frank Sinatra, Luciano Pavarotti, Mayor Daley, Marcel Marceau, and George Clooney. We ordered lasagna and a bottle of Chianti. I proposed a toast: "Here's to us." I felt like an "us" had emerged out of the unreal worlds of the museum and the funky old restaurant. Denise picked up the dinner tab. It had been her day.

By the end of the weekend, Denise casually informed me that she would like to see me again soon. I felt the same way. We started visiting each other, mostly in Kalamazoo, because she was working, and other than my school trips to San Francisco, I was free to see her in Michigan. When I arrived in the Kalamazoo airport, Denise would be waiting for me, jumping up and down with her arms up in the air like a cheerleader. During work days, I would stay in her home with Maddie, her black lab, and Hoshi, her tabby cat. I fixed breakfast each morning, and met her for lunch in Pfizer's cafeteria. I jogged each day and did my graduate work. We developed routines of living together. Denise was not only tolerant, she was easygoing. She cheered me up, not for a few moments, but in lasting ways that gave me lasting joy.

One day in mid-spring, we walked Maddie through a marshy nature preserve bordered by a lake covered with a thin layer of ice. Maddie, an old dog, lumbered out onto the ice and went through. Denise loved that dog. She screamed. In a rare show of heroism, I knocked a limb off a nearby tree, walked into the lake up to my thighs, and used the limb to beat on the ice to form a water path so Maddie could swim back to shore. I was a hero not only with Denise, but with Dana, and with John and Audrey.

Saving her dog may not have sealed the deal with Denise, but it didn't hurt. I still had the feeling she wasn't totally convinced that spending the rest of her life with me would be a good idea. She liked her independence.

Denise didn't especially need to get married. She was the kind of woman that both men and women liked. She had a ton of friends. Her mother and father lived a short distance away. Her father helped out with the handyman chores around the house that she owned. She had saved enough money for Dana's college education. People loved her at Pfizer. On Saturdays, she would buy a latte and do errands. Other times, she would go flying with her dad. On Sundays, she attended church. She started taking me to church on my weekend visits. She said that her mother had taught her how to be a Christian. She talked freely about her faith in God. We talked about trust. She had little trust in men. I realized that Denise needed to feel that I was completely devoted to her, and that she could count on me in every possible way.

As for me, I felt calm and peaceful around Denise. I began to form a faint outline of a new life together, one where we talked easily about everything, took longs walks with a dog, visited interesting places, and where we could appreciate and forgive each others' imperfections.

LESSON TWENTY-THREE

After a personal catastrophe, find someone to talk with every day, the way children and old people do.

24.

Once there, exhausted by the effort of the ascent,
My head pounding, lungs aching for air,
I sat down as soon as I could. My teacher said:
"Now would be a good time to stop being a
layabout."

Dante's Inferno, Canto XXIV

By the end of 2002, Saybrook had accepted my application for admission to their doctoral program in psychology. I thought that college teaching might be part of the answer to my question about how to spend the rest of my life. The most satisfying years of my life had been my school years. I loved to learn. So four months after Laurene died, I decided to begin a new chapter in my life.

The prospect of returning to the Bay Area excited me. Contrary to some of my friends in Texas, I loved the West Coast. I looked forward to once again sitting in the front row of a classroom and taking notes. I ordered my textbooks, and read the first one from beginning to end in one week. In March 2003, I attended student orientation. The schedule of residential and non-residential school work meant that I could remain in Houston, and not worry about selling the house.

Out of the Inferno

Our family gathered for the first time since Laurene's death in February. On February 14, 2003, Mom and Dad celebrated their 60th wedding anniversary. All four daughters were there, my brother and his family, and many friends. We had a fun ceremony at the Boca Royale Country Club in Englewood, Florida. The girls read some of their grandfather's love letters sent to Mom during the war, and brother Dave surprised everyone by playing "Always," Mom and Dad's favorite song, on my Dad's favorite musical instrument, the harmonica.

During the long drive back to Houston, I thought about how people's lives keep going after catastrophes—hurricanes, accidents, deaths, and after joyous events—weddings, anniversaries, birthdays, holidays, and graduations. Someone told me that Irene Brown, our guide during the visit to Brownwood, had died while traveling out-of-town to attend a friend's funeral. *Not a bad way to die. You travel to honor the living or the dead, to celebrate an important event, and you die in the process. Events and processes. The business of living well and dying well.*

I developed new friends during my first weeks at Saybrook University, a more diverse group than any I had encountered in my business career: an organization development professional from Yale, an engineer working for a high tech company in Silicon Valley, a Baptist preacher from Missouri, a family therapist from Seattle, a Mormon businessman from

Utah, a Jewish Buddhist professor from Berkeley, and a Latina business woman and social activist.

I joined a meditation group that met every day before breakfast. I learned mindfulness meditation and Yoga poses. In one session, we took turns hypnotizing each other. We learned about parapsychology, how normal people like me reported psychic experiences (like seeing your deceased wife appear), and other forms of extrasensory perception: telepathy, clairvoyance, precognition, and psychokinesis (moving objects with your mind).

I ate lots of new foods—chickpeas, tofu, hummus—and veggie potions reputed to have magical powers. I felt like I had been transported by Hogwarts Express to a Harry Potter World for adults. I thought about the radical differences between this curriculum and my first-year graduate business courses at Columbia: managerial accounting, elementary calculus, computer processing, statistical analysis, macroeconomics, and product marketing.

Even though the average Saybrook student took six years to complete a doctorate, I wanted to finish in three years. I figured out what I had to do. Before you could organize a dissertation committee, students had to complete two years of research methods courses. Since dissertations often took three years to complete, I could see how six years could pass without receiving a diploma. In addition to the methods courses, three

50-page pre-dissertation essays had to be completed and approved: one to critique a published dissertation in your field of interest, one to review literature relevant to your dissertation topic, and one to outline your research design.

It was possible to fast track some of the course work. If you finished all the requirements of a particular course, you could sign up for another course in the same semester. Unlike most of student colleagues who had full time work and families, I had no other responsibilities. I worked eight plus hours a day seven days a week. I had never been so enthused about anything in my life. The field of psychology fascinated me. The process of research intrigued me. After orientation week, I checked into a motel on the beach in Santa Cruz, and read hours every day. In addition to textbooks, each course required reading a foot-high stack of journal articles.

At work, people had jokingly nicknamed me "the professor." Others referred to me as Atom Ant, the geeky, sixties Hanna-Barbera cartoon character *("Up and At'em, Atom Ant!)*. Summoned by the police for difficult missions, Atom flew super speed like Batman to knock out bad guys like Ferocious Flea. In every episode, Atom Ant uses his smarts and strength to help people out. I had a tough-minded boss who called me "the social worker." The funny names people call you can end up becoming a hint about your true calling.

My first research course posed a critical question: how do you come up with ideas for research projects? During the evenings in Santa Cruz, I started thinking about topics. The earlier I identified an area of inquiry, the sooner I could organize my courses of study and ask professors with relevant backgrounds to sit on my dissertation committee. What topic did I care enough about to spend three years researching? Should I pick an organizational behavior topic from my business career, or did I have curiosities held over from the last ten years living close to breast cancer?

After mulling over topics for a couple weeks, I decided that I wanted to study the quality of life of long-term breast cancer survivors. I wanted to understand how cancer affects a person's overall sense of well-being over the course of their survivorship, their battle journey or journey battle. I also wondered how women with different socio-economic backgrounds and ethnicities experienced breast cancer. What parts of the difficult experience of coping with cancer were shared by all, and what parts were different based on race and ethnic background? This topic emerged as more important to me than anything else I considered. I wasn't ready to leave what had become my world.

During my first semester, I registered for a course titled HEALING AND RELATIONSHIPS.

Out of the Inferno

LESSON TWENTY-FOUR

When you run out of things to do, you may find what you were meant to do from the beginning—your true calling.

25.

Reader, if you find what I'm about to tell you
Hard to wrap your mind around, it's no wonder;
Even I who saw it can barely believe it.

Dante's Inferno, Canto XXV

After returning to Houston from Saybrook orientation, I received a call from a Dallas realtor named Howard. He represented Billy Connaway's property adjacent to the family farm in Brownwood. Just as Billy had told me, as soon as he passed away from heart failure, his family wanted to sell the land. On the way to Brownwood, I picked up a friend in College Station, a Texas A&M graduate, who knew a great deal about farm land management.

When we arrived in Brownwood, Ken and I walked Billy's property adjacent to Neil and Stella's old farm. Ken liked what he saw—swamp oaks, mature mesquite trees, a variety of grasses, heavy brush, and good drainage. I bought the property and a percentage of the mineral rights. My land acquisition tripled the size of Neil and Stella's homestead. I could see Neil smiling from heaven. *"Mighty fine!"* he would have said.

I drove Ken back to College Station, and then returned to Brownwood the next week. The land needed a new fence, and since I intended to lease the land for cattle, I also needed another water source. I took Delbert Connaway, another relation of Laurene's, out to breakfast at the Wagon Wheel in Brownwood. He introduced me to a man who happened to be eating breakfast in the same restaurant, not really a big coincidence in a small town. Edwin Cox. A bull dozer operator in his seventies, he had dozed out the first tank on Neil's property over thirty years before. In fact, he had been dozing land around Brownwood since he was sixteen. At the bottom of a draw near the lower end of the property, Cox dug a test hole. After drilling through 17 feet of soil, he hit gravel and rock.

"We can build more than a tank," he said. "That draw can hold a lake. Now, if you would like a like, you need to tell me how big. I charge $100 per hour, and I can build a small, medium, or large lake. A large lake would take about 100 hours and fill up in about six months, depending on the rain."

"A large lake," I said. "But what about permits?"

"Son, do you want a lake, or do you want to go to meetings?"

Two months later, I had a huge hole in the ground. I walked to the bottom and looked up and out of the earthy creation. Over the next six months, as Cox had said, intermittent rains slowly filled the hole with muddy water, like the opening of a large brown eye. You couldn't see the lake from the road, but you could see it from Google Earth. I had never done anything like this before. Contrary to the advice of the therapist who had pressed me to do nothing, I had supervised the creation of a beautiful home for birds and fish, and a source of water for cattle and wildlife.

I bought large plastic containers from a local feed store filled with a Noah's Ark of fish swimming in heavy duty plastic bags: minnows, blue gill, bass, and catfish. From the same store, I bought an automatic fish feeder to scatter seed over the water twice a day. I hired the local fence maker, who just as I had been told, scratched out an estimate based on a mule ride around the property line. When he had finished, a new six-strand barbed wire fence surrounded the combined farms, along with a front gate by the road, and another gate at the back. We preserved the original stone walls out of respect for history. As promised, Delbert talked the fence builder down on the price, and then Delbert leased the land from me for cattle production.

I kept going back to Brownwood. At one point, I thought I might build a house overlooking the lake. I liked the people in the area who often stopped by to talk on their way in to or out of town. One said, "Y'all ought to come live here. We have lots of rich widows up on pill hill." Walking behind the closed gates and fences, I felt protected from the outside world. I could also feel Neil's comforting presence ghosting around me in the fields and sitting beside me in a booth at Underwood's, his favorite restaurant. To this day, I can't rationalize why I bought the property other than for a beautiful refuge at a time in my life when I needed one. The psychologist had forewarned me about making impulse purchases. Oh, well.

***

I began research on a paper for my first research methods course. I wanted to study Laurene's breast cancer support group, Rosebuds. The group had been formed in January 1990, and over twelve years later, the group still thrived. Researchers were allowed, but on a limited basis. I wanted to identify success factors contributing to the long survival of the group, because my research showed that most support groups disband after three years. I gathered my information from one-on-one meetings with the participants and group leaders, and by reading the group's newsletters. This work tested whether or not I could handle interacting with breast cancer survivors considering what I had been through with over the last ten plus years. It didn't matter. I felt blessed to be working with these vital and vibrant women. And I felt engaged in useful work.

Rosebuds happened to be one of the first general breast cancer support groups in the Houston area, and is still going strong in 2016. In the beginning, so many women showed up for the meetings that they had to be divided into small circles to give everyone a chance to share. Certain norms developed: 1) listen more than offer advice, 2) it's okay to bring female friends or relatives, 3) membership is open to everyone, and 4) everything we discuss remains confidential. With these guidelines, women began to share their stories along with their emotions. There were mother/daughter participants, and women from various ethnic backgrounds and nationalities.

Over the years, other groups formed using rose as a metaphor based on the first name of Rose Kushner (1929-1990), a journalist who had been a pioneering advocate for breast cancer patients. The groups included: Rosebuds II for women for women with advanced breast cancer who wanted to share in ways that might have been too frightening or explicit in a larger group, *Las Rosas Vivas* for Latina women who felt more comfortable sharing with others from their own cultural background and in their native language, the Rose Garden, a general group like Rosebuds, for women living in the southeast area of Houston, and the Knockout Roses, a group for younger women (40 and under).

In 1994, Rosebuds leaders consulted with Karen Jackson, the founder of Sisters Network, when she was first forming a support group for African American women in Houston. (The Sisters Network eventually became a national organization with 40 chapters and 3,000 members.) In a number of cases, women attended more than one group. As I later discovered, while the groups had a lot in common, each group developed its own style to meet the needs of its members.

As I interviewed, I witnessed a beautiful unfolding of strength and love. Hearing the women talk, reminded me of Laurene's responses to a life-threatening illness. The women valued life. They wanted to beat the cancer. They needed support: information, opinions, social interaction, relaxation, and fun. The women also appreciated the privacy to discuss problems arising from treatment that were difficult to air with others, like spirituality, changes in sexuality, how to deal with mouth sores, and fears about dying. One woman said, "I showed another woman my mastectomy to help her decide whether to have one or not."

The organization of the group amazed me. A "doctor box" contained individual evaluations of oncologists and other specialists at MD Anderson. A "drug box" documented group member experiences with specific drugs to help women choose medications. The women reported on the availability of clinical trials. Participants had organized their particular backgrounds into specialties: finance, law, medical, complementary medicine, alternative therapy, management of side effects, website construction, newsletter writing, meeting warm-up activities, creation of a lending library, meeting facilitation, and community outreach activities like participation in "Race for the Cure."

These women were highly focused, and many had been referred to the group by their doctors. Attendance by outsiders was strictly limited in order to create a safe space to talk and listen. For example, vendors hawking reverse mortgages and other products could not attend. While most of the women in the group were white, two African American women attended, a Latina woman, and women from other countries including the Philippines and Pakistan. The women comprised a mix of rich and poor, professional and blue collar; women working, women not working, women looking for work. No men were allowed unless they had breast cancer. Spouses and children were not permitted, although they were included in activities outside the group meetings like picnics.

Discussion of co-existing conditions was limited. Also, the facilitators stressed that they were not a therapy group. Members who got off topic, or became dogmatic, or took too much air time, were reined in. The meeting descriptions sounded like business meetings to me: advance preparation, a meeting agenda, organized reporting, and accountabilities. The meetings started on time, and ended on time. One women laughed as she said, "If people want to chitchat, they can come before the meeting starts or stay afterwards."

My personal involvement in the project brought me back into familiar territory. Even though the group tried to focus on breast cancer and its immediate effects, I noticed how the larger issues outside the disease kept popping up: divorce, job loss, and other illnesses. Later when I was granted access to an actual meeting, I found the meeting to be less structured than advertised. There was a whole system of outside forces and relationships discussed, lots of chitchat and fun. In one meeting, the warm-up exercise involved sitting on a balloon until it popped, an antidote to the occasional doom and gloom ("We'll all be dead in three years.").

Giving back to part of the community who had supported Laurene and me for over ten years felt good. My professor commented that I was turning into a good scholar. I had never thought of myself as a scholar before. Most business people that I had known regarded academics with disdain. I observed that the people around me at Saybrook were doing worthwhile things, and creating new knowledge about people and the world, finding practical solutions to difficult problems.

Back to work! It felt good to be back at work. A new way of working. I'm sure Laurene is proud of me.

A Husband's Passage Through Cancerland

*There is something about breast cancer that I can do.
I need to hold on to my past. It wasn't all bad.*

LESSON TWENTY-FIVE

The path to healing might lead you back to the location of the original injury.

26.

...You've endured
Countless dangers to reach the west:
In the little time that's left
To feel something, don't deny yourselves
The chance to seek new life...

Dante's Inferno, Canto XXVI

In 2003, Dad's kidneys failed. He had developed nephritis shortly after the war, and his kidneys had given him problems throughout his adult life. He was feeling weak, but resolved to follow the rigors of dialysis. Just as Laurene had done, he decided to learn Spanish. He wanted to converse with his Latino dialysis technicians. I promised to bring him the textbook and learning guides that Laurene and I had used at the community college.

I flew from Houston to Sarasota for a visit. Dad was his usual cheerful self, but when I learned more of his medical regimen, I became concerned. Hemodialysis required many things to go well. He could not miss treatments. He had to follow a strict diet. He had to maintain the proper serum phosphate levels in his blood. Dad followed the instructions. I was still worried. He had experienced a heart attack in his sixties. His chronic kidney disease stemmed from a WWII injury, when he had suffered blunt force damage to his back from a kamikaze attack to his destroyer in the Battle of Leyte Gulf. He had been thrown up against a bulwark in the radar shack after a *kamikaze* loaded with an 1800-pound bomb missed the wheelhouse by twenty feet, crashing off the bow into the ocean.

I reviewed the Spanish workbooks with Dad while we sat together, the dialysis machine humming beside his bed. The clinic was full of patients arriving and departing from their appointments. They talked back and forth about their challenges with dialysis: transportation, absence of family support, cramping, feeling too bad or sick to make the appointments, and other medical conditions. Some of the patients talked and acted depressed. A typical statement, "What's the use? I'm going to die soon anyway." As for Dad, he loved machines. He learned how the dialyzers worked. For him, his appointments were like getting the car lubed and oiled. Mom was his major source of comfort and encouragement. The life expectancy of dialysis patients in the United States is the lowest in the industrialized world. Based on Dad's age, the median survival was 1.3 years. Dad wanted to live for another ten years. His resolve reminded me of Laurene.

While in Florida, I longed for Denise. At the same time, I felt guilty about falling in love with another woman so soon after Laurene's death (what would the children say?). I asked myself how I could love a woman who in many ways was very different from Laurene. Denise was more like me. Had I come to a point in my life where I was happy enough with me to find a partner closer to my own personality? What was it about Denise that engendered a longing to be with her? Was loneliness driving me prematurely into the arms of another woman, or was my love for Denise real? And if I moved too fast, would I scare her away? Would she question my motives? "Don't date for at least a year," the psychologist had said.

I knew that Laurene was still present for me. I realized that I talked to Denise too much about Laurene, and sometimes I called Denise Laurene by mistake. She said she didn't mind, but she probably did mind. I kept thinking of our telephone conversation after our breakfast meeting in Kalamazoo: "What do you like about me?" I could now do better than comment on her eyes. I liked her competence with so many things I wasn't any good at, her wide range of interests, her optimism, her warmth, her empathy, her adaptability, her popularity with both men and women, her love of animals, and her vivid imagination.

A few weeks later, I flew back to Florida again to be with Mom and Dad. Dad wasn't doing well. Denise happened to be in Tampa visiting her sister. Debby's brain tumor had continued to grow despite two surgeries. The doctors were considering experimental treatments. I asked Denise if she would like to meet my parents before she returned to Michigan. She arrived in a rental car the next day, and we spent the afternoon together. After visiting with Mom and Dad, we took a walk on a nature trail in the neighborhood. Denise wanted to talk about her sister, and I wanted to talk about Dad. After a half hour, I decided to let her know how I felt about her. I told her that I loved her. She said that she loved me too. Rather than asking me what I liked about her, this time, she asked what I didn't like about her.

I knew I had to be honest. Denise had the strongest bullshit detector that I had ever experienced in a man or woman. I also knew she was a highly sensitive person. Since she took me by surprise, I had no time to think, so I started on safe ground.

"I like everything about you," I said.

"That's not an acceptable answer," she said. "Now tell me."

"Well, you don't like loud, unexpected noises, so I have to be careful not to startle you."

"You'll have to do better than that."

"When you make mistakes, you take it personally.

"I never make mistakes, but go on."

"You don't like to see violent movies."

"True that, go on."

"You don't trust men."

"I might trust you...tell me more."

"You're bossy," I said.

This is the part where I thought I had gone too far. Denise's eyes looked up and sideways. She hunched her shoulders, and bowed her head with a *I-did-something-wrong-look* on her face. Had I struck home, or was she exercising her flair for drama? Her lips quivered a bit too long. She broke out in a smile, followed by a raised eyebrow of fake anger.

"You need supervision," she replied with a sweet smile.

I could never match Denise's facial expressions, but I must have given her a *what-am-I-going-to-say-next?* look. She smothered me with hugs and kisses. The inquisition had ended. We finished our walk holding hands. We walked at the same pace.

After Denise left for the airport, I drove to St. Armand's Circle in Sarasota to buy a chocolate ice cream cone and an engagement ring. I knew I had more work to do to win over Denise. I had to choose the right place to ask her to marry me, a place surrounded by fantasy and romance. Denise was a story-book girl at heart.

LESSON TWENTY-SIX

There is no right time to fall in love.

27.

When I reached that inevitable stage in life
When one should, as they say, bring down their sails
And gather ropes,
...I repented, confessed, and chose to serve—

Dante's Inferno, Canto XXVII

Latina women and their children filled the room with rapid conversation and laughter. Cancer survivors routinely attended with friends and family—mothers, grandmothers, aunts, girlfriends, and hordes of children, all speaking Spanish. *Las Rosas Vivas* (the living roses) created a family atmosphere of kindness, friendliness, and respect. But a key part of the family was missing—men. As the meeting progressed, I found out why. Everyone spoke Spanish, so I was happy to have a bi-lingual doctor of internal medicine with me who translated. I am certain that in addition to cultural affinities, the Latina women were comfortable attending a meeting in their native language. For those who did not speak English, it was a necessity.

As the meeting opened, I could tell that these women were plain scared. They had little information about breast cancer and treatment options. The Latina women in the room represented thirteen different countries. Only a few of the women were multi-lingual, and few were American citizens. So beyond basic lack of knowledge, access to medical care predominated the conversations. Getting into clinical trials was nearly impossible. One undocumented woman said, "We don't ask questions, because we're afraid what questions will be asked us." A Latina social worker who attended the meetings reported on her attempts to help the women find doctors, and navigate the health care system. It was not easy.

Another source of fear stemmed from culture. Some believed that you could catch cancer. Another woman said, "We don't believe you are sick until symptoms appear, and then it's too late." In addition to fatalism and fear, other cultural barriers kept crept into the meeting. For example, when discussing the difficulties of attending support group meetings, one said, "*La ropa sucia se lava en casa*" (we wash our dirty laundry in our houses). Another said, "We don't talk about our breasts."

Other women mentioned that attending the meetings required overruling their husbands, who expected them to stay home and do the cooking and other family chores. The isolation of these women outside a few family and friends rose to the foreground as the meetings continued: "I have no one to talk to, my people are all in South America," one woman said.

Other comments revealed a mistrust of health care providers, including a mistrust of physicians (only about 12% of the doctors in the US are Hispanic). This discussion made me think why these women had formed their own group, rather than melding into a culturally diverse group where more resources would be available. As the meeting drew near an end, I had my answer. With the help of my translator, I wrote down what one Latina woman said, "It is difficult to share with people outside our culture." she said. "We have a common language, and we need to share our emotions."

After attending this meeting, I decided that my dissertation research had to be more than an academic exercise. My heart was touched by the suffering on the faces of these women. And the fear. Their family oriented culture and their ease in expressing their emotions, however, added a needed strength to cancer survivorship. It was abundantly clear to me that in both sickness and health, a Latina woman could not live without the love and support of her family. While this was not unique to the Hispanic culture, family orientation stood out every time I met with these women, as a central focus and a cultural strength.

I concluded that the three ethnic groups (African American, Latina, and white women) could learn from each other. While I saw similar behavior across groups around support and caring for each other, each group possessed strengths that seem to be rooted in the cultural backgrounds of the participants. There appeared to be important differences with respect to self-advocacy, family support, and community involvement. I contacted my dissertation advisers, and changed my research method to participative action research. I wanted not only to describe change, but help create it.

A month later, I convened the first meeting of what later became SHARE Houston Breast Cancer Support Group Network. Support group leaders came up with the SHARE acronym: Support, Hope, Awareness, Respect, Empowerment). We started with five support groups, and later added others. There were more breast cancer support groups in Houston than I had imagined. The next group to join was composed of Chinese-speaking women. The group of Chinese women was followed by a group comprised of breast cancer survivors diagnosed with breast cancer at age 40 or younger.

We met each month for lunch in the Cleburne Cafeteria on Bissonnet Street near MD Anderson. Creating and distributing information on breast cancer hotlines and support groups surfaced as the first priority. Once established, support group leaders began to make cross-referrals where groups other than their own might be more helpful to a particular individual. We shared best practices in group facilitation. The Network eventually expanded to include groups in West Houston, Central Houston, and South Houston—the network mushroomed from members of twenty-two support groups.

The leaders of these groups guided my research. They opened doors for me. They suggested how to alter my research design. They turned out to be my personal board of directors through the next three years. These women validated the usefulness of what I was attempting. They made me feel important again by serving their needs. We began to discover the relative cultural strengths represented by the diverse set of support groups; for example, the individualism and self-responsibility of white women, the emotional and family support of Latina women, and the spiritual and community support of African American women.

Rather than reaching for a bannister while descending a staircase to old age, I was stepping up in the world as a scholar and community servant—giving back rather than giving up. I had also surrounded myself with the support of literally hundreds of brave and beautiful women.

Thank you, God.

LESSON TWENTY-SEVEN

If you're missing support in dealing with tough challenges like cancer, see what you can learn from what works in cultures other than your own.

28.

Hearing that, over a hundred stopped suddenly
To stare at me in awe,
Forgetting for a moment their agony.

Dante's Inferno, Canto XXVIII

I had never heard a black woman pray. I was sitting in the back of a large community room in the New Faith Baptist Church, a half hour's drive southwest of downtown Houston, on a Saturday morning. The church is huge, serving over 2,000 families. The monthly meeting of the Sisters Network began with a prayer that would last fifteen minutes. I counted fifty women. The content, cadence, thoughts, and emotions that the pastor expressed stirred me to the level of religious experience. Her voice boomed full, rich, deep, and powerful.

I could tell that God had touched her in ways that I could only imagine. She left no stone unturned. She prayed for everyone in the room, many by name. She prayed for me, the white guy in the back that everyone had glanced at once or twice. The Old and New Testaments contributed to the phrasing of her statements of gratitude and praise. She prayed to God, Jesus, and the Holy Spirit. If there had been a test of Christian principles after the prayer, anyone who was listening could have aced the test.

Out of the Inferno

Hymns followed that I knew from my Methodist upbringing. I thought, this is more of a church service than a support group meeting. After the prayers and singing, every single woman stood up to give a short report. One woman said, "I've lost 250 pounds since the last meeting." She paused while every one gasped. "I dumped my husband. He wasn't being helpful, so I dumped him." Applause and laughter followed. Some of the individual reports were more like affirmations: "I know in my heart that I am healed," "I am debt free," "I have a closer relationship with God," "I know what my body needs to be healthy." There were also reports on two women who had passed away since the last meeting. Many of the Sisters had attended her memorial service.

Next there was a warm-up activity. Every woman present was asked to parade her shoes across the front of the room, and tell why she had worn those particular shoes that day. I noticed that all the women wore beautiful dresses and head scarves. Their decisions about what shoes to wear was comical and entertaining. I relaxed and started to enjoy myself until the facilitator invited me to the front of the room to parade my shoes. Everyone cheered me to the front. No longer an outsider taking notes, I was inserted front and center into the meeting. I was wearing plain old black tie shoes. I can't remember what I said, but everyone thought what I said was funny, or maybe they laughed because a white man was up in front of

50 black women talking about how he chooses to dress.

From the committee reports that followed, the community orientation of this group became evident. Breast cancer was not an individual concern or a concern confined to a particular family, but a full blown concern of Houston's Fifth Ward. The women held fundraisers, organized block walks to sign women up for mammograms, and in addition to supporting the families of deceased members, they organized parties to celebrate birthdays and anniversaries. Husbands and children came in and out of the room, but did not attend the meetings. You could hear the constant banter of people walking by the open door, and the pounding of basketballs on the courts down the hall.

At the end of the meeting, a number of women responded to my request for individual tape-recorded interviews. I received positive responses to similar requests from the Rosebuds and *Las Rosas Vivas.* In the following weeks, my initial observations were confirmed through one-on-one interviews that lasted up to two hours each. As I replayed the tape recordings and reviewed my notes, I drew some tentative conclusions. My overall impression was that Rosebuds had an individual focus, *Las Rosas Vivas,* a family focus, and Sisters Network, a community focus.

At this early stage in the research process, I wanted to see if the data from my interviews supported these initial observations. Over the next three years, I entered 870 interview quotes into a database. With help from my statistics professor, I performed a chi-square analysis of over 21,000 word choices. White women most often used *my story* to describe their cancer experiences, and used more personal pronouns like *I* and *me* than women from the other groups. The stories of the Latina women were laced with references to *my people, my family,* or *in my house.* Black women summarized their experiences as *my witness* or *my testimony,* accompanied by frequent references to *God* and *community.*

The differences across the groups were statistically significant, even though the actual data from my interviews was highly nuanced. For example, the individualistic style of the Rosebuds did not mean that the women were self-centered. In fact, I discovered numerous examples of how Rosebuds not only helped members within the support group, but reached out to breast cancer patients and survivors outside their circle. One of the Rosebuds received a grant from the National Cancer Institute (and later two Department of Defense grants) to develop culturally appropriate educational materials for both African American and Latina groups. Another Rosebud, an immigration lawyer, helped a Brazilian woman get a visa for her mother.

Latina women used the word "we" twice as often as black women, and three times more often than white women. Latina women used a family related word once out of every 100 words, a statistically significant difference from the other two groups. This family orientation of Latina women was not a singular blessing. Many Latina women had tremendous obstacles to overcome from husbands who refused to alter their lives in the slightest to help their wives manage breast cancer. The challenges ranged from housework to sex. Other family members ostracized Latina women, because they assumed that breast cancer was caused by some kind of moral failure.

Black women used "God" or "Almighty" three to five times more often than the other two groups, and "work" was used five to ten times more often than the other two groups. More black women worked than the other groups, because they had to work out of necessity, although "poor" women attended all three groups. Most of these working women held down full time jobs before, during, and after their cancer treatment. As with the other groups, cultural orientation turned out to have both positive and negative aspects. For African American women, trust in God proved to be a mixed blessing in that some women trusted that God would completely take care of them, and did nothing on their own behalf. Some even refused treatment. Women who viewed God as a partner on their breast cancer journey seemed to have better medical outcomes.

So the data did not fall into neat categories, because the women had developed personal strategies for dealing with breast cancer that cut across any generalizations about them. Also, white women attended Sisters meetings, African American and Latina women attended Rosebuds, and some women attended more than one group.

The week after I attended the Sisters meeting, I received a call from ninety-year-old Gladys, a fifty-year breast cancer survivor. "We're so glad you attended last Saturday. We hope you come again." As she continued before I could get a word in, I gathered she thought I was a woman who with breast cancer. Rather than jumping in to correct her, I let her finish. I'm glad I did. The love and gentleness of her words were heartfelt. Finally, she paused for me to respond.

"I was the white guy in the back of the room," I said. "You know, the one with black shoes."

"After each meeting we call all the people who signed in. Now I know who you are...your wife passed on, and you decided to help folks like us."

LESSON TWENTY-EIGHT

If you listen to what other people say about who you are from their perspective, you may redefine your life work.

29.

*"...The moon is already below us;
We'll soon have used up the little time we've been given
And there's more to see than this.*

Dante's Inferno, Canto XXIX

Denise loved Jane Austen. She belonged to the Jane Austen Society. She had read all of Austen's novels multiple times, including the annotated editions. She had dvd's of the movie versions of all the Jane Austen movies and television adaptions. Tears would form in her (brown) eyes when she watched Elizabeth accept Darcy's proposal in the 1995 BBC version. She read the novels over and over again, and re-watched the movies. She was interested in costume design and loved the period costumes. In college, she had sketched costumes for drama productions.

A number of her relatives had been in the movie business. Aunt Dorothy Short and Uncle Dave O'Brien had starred in numerous movies in the 1930s, including the cult movie, *Reefer Madness,* a melodrama about high school students who are lured by pushers to try marijuana (the original title: *Tell Your Children).* During the movie, Aunt Dorothy gets fatally shot because of a pot-induced hallucination.

Uncle Dave starred in a number of low-budget Westerns, but is best known as "Captain Midnight," a movie serial actor. Madeline Talcott, her aunt, played a bit role in *The Raven* (1935) starring Boris Karloff. Diane, Denise's oldest sister, had lived and acted in New York City, and was now a Hollywood agent working out of a ranch house in Montana. She had fallen in love with a cowboy whom she met in a bar, THE ROAD KILL CAFE, during the filming of *A River Runs Through It*.

Denise had drama in her blood, and romance in her heart. How could I do something bigger than life to close the deal? I had the engagement ring, but did I have the right stuff to make her happy? Would she turn down my marriage offer, as Elizabeth had first turned down Darcy? When I graduated from high school, she had been ten years old. She was a lot more animated and fun than me. I needed to show her that I could do something special, something with uncustomary flair. I didn't want her to repeat what she had said after our breakfast in Kalamazoo: "I'm not your type." I wanted to organize every detail of a true adventure that would impress her enough to marry me.

So here was my plan. I organized a Jane Austen tour of England. We would meet in London. Denise said she could book a Virgin Atlantic flight out of Kalamazoo through Newark. I took a Houston/Newark itinerary with United. I arrived at a posh hotel in London on schedule, but Denise's flight was delayed. I picked her up at Heathrow the next day. Her bags wouldn't arrive until three days later—not a great start. Denise purchased some basic clothes on Jermyn Street, and I lent her a few shirts and sweaters. I made a few adjustments in our itinerary, but I forged ahead with determination to implement my grand plan. At least Denise seemed to be upset with Virgin Atlantic rather than me.

We drove a rental car two hours to the Cotswold's. I took three paper map guides with me titled *The Cotswold's by Car 1,2, and 3*. Denise navigated and I drove, managing to operate the stick shift with my left hand, and turn in the right (left) direction on the roundabouts. We enjoyed finding all the quaint towns and points of interest. The land was beautiful in autumn. We passed through village greens enlivened by small streams, parish churches fronting churchyards filled with old gravestones, stands of beech trees, and every now and then, we watched a pheasant or a partridge cross the narrow roads in front of us.

Near the town of Stow-on-the-Wold and a quarter mile from the village of Lower Codington (not far from Upper Codington), we found a small country church built in the 12th century. Inside we found medieval wall paintings. Later in the day, the wind picked up and it started to rain, but we persisted to find the Roll right Stones, a circle of Neolithic and

Bronze Age megaliths described by legend as a monarch and his courtiers petrified by a witch.

That evening, November 17, 2003, we stayed at Bribery Court Hotel, an old stone manor house on the edge of the Cotswold's. We sat down by a fire to enjoy an aperitif before dinner and look at the menus. Bad news arrived. Debby had lost her battle with brain cancer. After we left for our trip, she had taken a sudden turn for the worse. Diane had flown to Florida from Montana, and sat beside her at the hospital. Diane called us to say that Debby had passed away, a beautiful woman in her early fifties taken away by cancer one year to the day after I had lost Laurene.

The next morning, Denise and I went into an old stone chapel on the grounds of the manor house, and improvised a memorial service for Debby. We prayed, and walked slowly around the vacant sanctuary to read about the lives of men and women inscribed in plaques on the stone walls. We walked through the ancient graveyard outside. Denise and Debby had been close. Now my dream trip had been marred not only by temporary inconveniences, but by a terrible personal loss. With Debby's memorial service set after our scheduled return, we decided to keep going. The next day, we checked out of the hotel and headed to Bath, the next stop on our Jane Austen tour.

On the flight to England, I had read *Northanger Abbey,* the first of Jane Austen's novels to be completed for publication. Jane Austin died in July, 1817, and the book was published in late December, 1817. In the novel, Catherine Morland, one of ten children of a country clergyman, travels to Bath at the invitation of wealthy neighbors. Catherine was to partake in the winter season balls, theater, and other social activities. Denise and I visited the huge ballrooms, and the Jane Austen Center which houses an exhibition of the six years (1801-1806) Jane Austin stayed in Bath. We had afternoon tea.

We spent two days in Bath before setting out for the village of Lacock where I had planned my proposal at the very spot where Darcy had proposed to Elizabeth in the BBC movie. Only one minor problem. I didn't know where the very spot happened to be. Certainly the villagers would know.

Lacock, with its grid of four streets, sits on Bide Brook, a stream that runs north to the Avon River. An Iron Age camp and a Roman road lie a half mile to the south of the village. The town remains much as it looked in the eighteenth century—timber-framed stone and brick houses with weathered stone roof tiles encrusted by lichen and moss. You could imagine the town two hundred years ago, alive with markets and fairs, peddlers and sideshows, animals and poultry in front of the shops and businesses. We decided to have lunch at the Red Lion on High Street. I planned to make a stealth move. While Denise looked for the restroom, I approached some elderly men at the bar to ask for directions. These were the villagers that I had in mind. The locals would know everything. They might even draw me a map.

I pointed to the restroom. "I'm going to propose marriage to that lady after lunch."

"You're making a mistake, sir," an older man said. "I tried marriage once, and I must say it leaves much to be desired."

"I'm going to go ahead and ask her, but I need your help. I want to find the place where BBC filmed the TV version of *Pride and Prejudice*, around 1994 or 1995."

The men sitting at the bar engaged in a brief but vigorous argument about where I should go, but by the time Denise returned to our table, I had verbal directions. We finished lunch. As Denise headed to the door, I gave the chief bar spokesman a whisper:

"I'll come back later and tell you how I did," I said.

"Don't bother, we won't be here. Never spend more than one hour in a one pub. We'll be somewhere else by then, another pub."

As instructed, Denise and I walked down High Street to East Street. We passed the massive timbers of a 14th-century tithe barn, and the village hall. We approached the high-arched 15th-century Lacock Church. At the end of East Street by a bakery, we turned and followed a footpath to a large meadow. We climbed over a stone style, walked around some cows, crossed a footbridge over a small brook, and arrived at our destination (or close enough I thought). We had arrived in the middle of a footpath between two small villages, a path bordered by a black stone fence and overhanging trees. A brook sparkled in the field below us. Birds filled the fields. I had rehearsed the famous words of Darcy's (Colin Firth) proposal to Elizabeth (Jennifer Ehle):

"You are too generous to trifle with me. If your feelings are still what they were last April, tell me so at once. *My* affections and wishes are unchanged, but one word from you will silence me on this subject forever."

But I thought that might be a bit overdone, so I simply said, "Denise, will you marry me?"

"Yes," she answered. She cried. For the first time since we had been dating, she cried. I cried, too.

We took a selfie with my camera.

Pride and Prejudice continues:

"They walked on, without knowing in what direction. There was so much to be thought, and felt, and said, for the attention of any other objects."

In our case, one of us walked on, without knowing in what direction. Denise knew exactly where we were going.

Once we found the car and for our return to London, I made a wrong turn, and drove thirty miles in the wrong direction. Denise took charge of the map, and she has never let me read a map again. Just as she had guided me through the Museum of Science and Industry in Chicago, she had taken on the larger job of guiding me through life. She was right. I need supervision!

LESSON TWENTY-NINE

Love and loss are universal and unlimited.

30.

"You, who are inexplicably in this miserable world—
Without being punished—
Take a good long look," he said.

Dante's Inferno, Canto III

"Let's start with your research hypothesis."

"I don't have one yet."

"Didn't they tell you to start with a research hypothesis in the methods course?"

"I didn't do it that way."

"That way is called the scientific method."

"I know, but I thought if I started with the raw data, the hypothesis would emerge."

"You've designed the research backwards."

"People call it grounded research—you come up with a theory by analyzing data."

"Sounds like the scientific method turned upside down."

"Well, I have lots of data."

I sat in a chair in my Houston home, and listened to three years of taped interviews. At my suggestion, the women had given themselves assumed names for the dissertation: Betsy, Kate, Prez, Louise, Ruth, Figbee, Susie Q, Dorothy, Esperanza, Clavelle, Estrella, Luna, Violeta, Kari, Estela, Elizabeth, and so on. Most of the women had shared a story behind their name choice. Some of the names represented friends or relatives, some names stood for their aspirations and hopes, other names were whimsical and made us laugh. How could I fit what I heard into the straight jacket outline of a scholarly dissertation?

I listened until after midnight, night after night. I soon realized that there was something going on with me beyond the rational research process. I kept playing the interviews over, because the women's stories brought Laurene back to me. I realized that at some level, my selection of the dissertation topic had been a way of keeping Laurene alive. The words reminded me of similar situations that Laurene and I had encountered. In some cases, the words were the same: "I will not let cancer rob me of my joy," "I refuse to have cancer define my life." The interviews also reminded me that the world after Laurene was not empty, but filled with other lives struggling to find meaning and hope in the middle of pain, suffering, and disappointment.

After weeks of sorting and categorizing, a new state of being developed in me. I felt transcended beyond the task at hand, like I was approaching the sacred in the middle of the crowd of data. For both survivors and caregivers, I began to see breast cancer as a life-changing event embedded with both positive and negative qualities. As I listened to the interviews, I was struck by how survivors engaged in a process of holding on and letting go to attitudes, beliefs, and ways of living as they developed their own unique responses to breast cancer. On the survivorship road, the survivors moved towards a destination that brought them into a closer connection with their true selves, with other people, with their community, and with their God. With every step, they suffered, but kept on going.

Once I developed general categories, I kept reworking the data into subcategories. A model of breast cancer survivorship blossomed before me like a flower that had only needed a little soil, sun, and rain. The model divided into three parts: 1) MY ROAD, 2) MY WALK, AND 3) MY DESTINATION. Each of these major categories contained personal strategies that moved survivors along what one black woman described as the zig-zag road, and a Latina woman called *mis andanzas* or my wanderings.

MY ROAD included all the givens that breast cancer survivors had to deal with: 1) cultural context, 2) stage of survivorship, 3) unique personal experiences, and 4) how they related to friends, family, community, God and Nature (what I called their other orientation).

Cultural context included research participant comments about how well they were adjusted to their surroundings. Recent immigrants, for example, had spent most of their lives living in other countries, and lacked basic knowledge of what resources might be available. Language barriers compounded the problem. Cultural context also included comments about beliefs, income, education, race, and ethnicity. For example, white women looked at the support group as a "virtual mother," black women described the "instant sisterhood" that accompanied a breast cancer diagnosis, and Latina women said they needed to talk about "dirty laundry," subjects that could not be discussed inside or outside their homes, especially their fears, shame, and ignorance about breast cancer.

Racism and prejudice presented many obstacles to African American and Latina women in terms of inequitable health care facilities and access to services. One black woman described a meeting with a doctor: "He says, 'I can't cut corners for you. The hospital won't allow me to cut corners for you. So you need to get a job. You can wait three months. Just go and get a job and some insurance...and then we can do everything okay, because the hospital is not going to let me do everything that I can do.'"

More than overt acts, these women were concerned about lack of affinity with their doctors and other caregivers, and they did not trust the system to support their best interests. Distrust also stemmed from conflicts between what women heard from doctors and nurses and culturally-based information: "cancer is fatal," "cancer is contagious," "cancer is shameful," "cancer is a punishment," "cancer is God's will," "nothing can be done."

MY ROAD inevitably included the stages of survivorship. Newly-diagnosed women wanted information and physician support above all else. An overwhelming need for decision-making information on treatment options dominated their attention. Gaining the support of family, friends, support groups, and other women with breast cancer experience dominated the data.

Women at the next survivorship stage (in most cases, the year after initial treatment) expressed the challenge of living a "new normal" life. As I listened to the tapes, the dampened down mood, tone, and feeling of the comments gave me the impression of a let down. Some women felt like the love and attention they had received in their first year lessened once the emergency had ended. Some felt numbed after the immediate coping with the diagnosis ceased, like digging out after a terrible hurricane had passed. Others felt that the health care system had dropped them. Fear of recurrence also lurked in the background—what one woman called fear of the *"the big whammy."*

For women with advanced disease, integrating spirituality into everyday life surfaced. Black women strengthened their faith with support from their church communities, Latina women felt that God accompanied them throughout their lives and held firm to their religious beliefs and practices. Many women were more likely to see spirituality as a complement to good medicine, and would only turn their lives over to God when all else failed.

While there was much in common, each woman in the research group had a unique story of their inner life with advanced disease. Some remained realistic and clinical until the end, actively resistant, pushing against obstacles; using their skills and talents to assert control over cancer, and to preserve their dignity. Other women would gain strength and lose strength over time, and eventually learned to care for themselves through all the ups and downs of living, losing, thriving, surviving. Use of alternative and complementary medicine increased with advanced disease. One of the women said, "My life has been fuller, richer, deeper, and more powerful than before cancer."

In addition to differences in personal experience, I heard how the survivorship process played out with different orientations—the individual, family, and community cultural anchors.

White women tended to show a strong individual orientation. They focused on the future, prized individual achievement, and saw themselves as dominant in how they related to the natural world. White women talked about special diets, travel plans, exercise regimens. One even developed a five-year plan. One said, "We all fall down and get up." Another, "You have to learn how to be a self-advocate." Other comments: "I can beat this," "You have to be strong," "I find my own path, my own resources, " "I need to do this on my own," "When I was diagnosed, neither my husband nor my religion helped, so I decided to go to for counseling." One of my favorites from a woman who traveled the world after her diagnosis, "I'm going to make sure the next Mrs. _____ doesn't spend my hard-earned money."

Latina women lived in a world of family. In some case, family members were obstacles. More often than not, Latinas were required to maintain their traditional roles and responsibilities through treatment. Their attempts to live in new ways were often thwarted by these expectations. The family orientation still provided the greatest source of support for them—for sympathy, friendship, respect, and loyalty. They surrounded themselves with their families, and brought family members to doctor's appointments and to support group meetings.

Black women lived in the world of a faith community. "God won't put on me more than I can bear," one woman said. "Keep hope and have faith," was the motto. Beyond faith, the overall community orientation of black women was evident in these comments: "We take care of people in our community," "We have block walks where we pound on doors in the Fifth Ward and get people to local churches for mammograms and breast cancer awareness sessions," "Being in a group helps you live longer," "I want to give back by helping others."

My initial impressions about ethnic and cultural differences were confirmed as my research continued, as well as the need to learn from the best that other cultures offered. White women needed more connection to their families, the community, and spiritual strength. Latina and black women needed access to the technical information, health care delivery systems, and specialized medical expertise that were more easily accessible to white women.

THE ROAD, or list of givens, also included personal experiences or conditions. Many women had other illnesses along with breast cancer, like chronic fatigue syndrome, diabetes, or heart disease. Divorce and other forms of family estrangement were factors. Women had different reactions to changes in their bodies: "I chose to be bald," "I hated to look at myself in the mirror." Age, energy, physical conditions, and clinical outcomes contributed to the personal experience of breast cancer beyond the shared experience. As I aggregated the data, I had to be careful not to lose what I could learn from the individual stories, often expressed in mottos. A Latina woman's motto: *"Cada día me siento sana, feliz y contena illena de felicidad y alegría. Ja Ja Ja!"* (Every day I feel healthy, happy, content, full of happiness and joy. Ha, Ha, Ha!*).*

A few weeks later, I called my dissertation adviser with two after-the-fact research questions: 1) Can a model of breast cancer quality of life be developed that accurately describes the lived experience of breast cancer survivors, and 2) can such a model help survivors improve the quality of their lives? I stuck the statement in the "research problem" section of my dissertation introduction.

My adviser had been right. I did the whole thing backwards. The model had developed out of what the women had told me. If I had laid out my research questions in advance, they would have probably been the wrong questions.

I know I'm not a great navigator, but I often find treasures while wandering around lost. My research process had followed the path that Latina women had used to describe their journey with breast cancer— *andanza,* a personal way of moving through the world, an adventure unique to each human being, the way you know how the people you love walk. I finally understood why these women had described living with breast cancer as *andanza* rather than *caminar*, the more common word for walk. By listening to the stories of hundreds of women over three years, I had created something original, a result more important than proving scholarly proficiency or meeting academic requirements.

LESSON THIRTY

We can learn from the experience of others who have lived with long-term illnesses.

31.

We turned our backs on the miserable valley
And climbed the bank that encircles it...
Here it wasn't as dark as night but still
Not light as day, so I couldn't see very far
  ahead...

Dante's Inferno, Canto XXXI

As the model of survivorship emerged from the data, THE WALK *(andanza)* followed THE ROAD. THE WALK summarized personal strategies women employed as they embarked on their particular breast cancer adventures or wanderings. I could quickly divide this category into two subcategories: HOLDING ON and LETTING GO. These alternating strategies had an overall sense of direction about them that lead to the final category of the model: DESTINATION. The path looked like the evasive zig-zag maneuvers Dad's World War II destroyer had taken through the sea to avoid enemy submarines, action often taken at night without running lights through dangerous waters with reefs and shoals.

Life for cancer survivors was not considered a linear progression from birth through death. The death of the former self left a new self. The old normal attitudes and behaviors and beliefs that had been perfectly serviceable before cancer were found deficient. Body image changed. Physical and mental capabilities changed. Relationships changed, and new relationships formed. The ebb and flow of daily life altered in large and small ways. In a moment's time after hearing the word *malignant,* women had to reconstruct their worlds, and grieve the death and dying of part of themselves. They had to experiment and improvise rather than rely on traditions, precedents, and past practices. One woman described the THE WALK as more like navigating "permanent white water."

Laurene let go of her business career, but held on to her family and friends. She left projects unfinished, plans incomplete, and a to do list with actions unfinished or scratched off. What she valued most remained. She could no longer be a perfectionist. She no longer needed to indulge me by learning how to play golf. Her self-concept could no longer be defined by what she hoped to become, the things she most dearly wanted for herself, like becoming a grandmother. She would have to let go of her idea that life is fair, and accept that circumstances don't always turn out they way one thinks they should.

Everything she had gained in her life would have to be relinquished, both what she produced and what the world thought of it. She could no longer delay coming to terms with unquestioned beliefs and assumptions. She would have to die with the record of what she had been. She could focus on only the most important matters in front of her: how to say goodbye, how to enjoy last pleasures, how to transcend her mind and body, how to die with dignity, how to be alone in the face of death. She had to let go of becoming the special case at the tail end of a probability distribution. She had to let go of a world of facts and clarity and consistency for a world of mystery and confusion and messiness.

The HOLDING ON and LETTING GO statements from the research participants seemed like a competition between life and death: the desire to hold on to a tenuous and temporary life, and to prolong an independent existence versus the pain and suffering, and the inescapable reality of death. These statements contained less glossing over than other statements. The statements seemed more practical and conveyed a willingness to accept reality as is. The statements reflected tough choices about how to spend increasingly valuable time. The image came to mind of two people tugging on either end of a rope, with one person saying, "Give it to me, I want it," and the other saying, "No, it's mine."

HOLDING ON/LETTING GO comments:

I made a list of all the things I loved, and then noted how much time I spent each day doing these things. I stopped commuting two hours each day to work, and moved my office to my home.

When I help others, I relax.

I gave up my job at an oil company to become a medical librarian.

I continued to work.

I began to let people help me, rather than turning down their offers.

When things get really bad, I hibernate.

Every day after work, I meditate for an hour.

You have to wait for the healing.

The support group let me cry all I wanted to.

God is going to take care of me.

I feel a lot of gratitude for being alive.

Sometimes I need to be still.

I surrendered all.

The less active LETTING GO activities made room for the more active HOLDING ON activities in much the same way as a weather front creates a low pressure area giving room for the next front to advance, never forming more than a brief equilibrium.

One woman described hitting a brick wall of opposing forces when she could not discuss cancer with her family. Attending support group meetings helped her talk about her breast cancer, and eventually she brought her family into the discussion, and drew them closer to her.

Another woman talked about holding on and letting go of fear:

"I moved away from horror, fear, and shame to feeling blasé and numb. When I found out there were no positive lymph nodes, I thanked God, and began to focus on taking care of my children, and attending support group meetings."

MY DESTINATION *(mi destino)* described an eventual sense of having arrived at a place of integration and peace. When Laurene said that she had been loved as a way of summing up her life, she had arrived at a destination. Other women talked about finding self and others, finding community, feeling safe, or restoring balance. The tones of voices from my individual and group interviews communicated a feeling of surrender and also of triumph. There was a sense of integration or wholeness; an expanded awareness or transcendence, like the women had let go of a more limited world view and were now holding on to an expanded, higher-order view of themselves and the world.

DESTINATION comments:

I have peace.

I have learned to take care of myself first, and then I take care of others.

I am realizing some of my dreams.
I'm going to Heaven with Jesus.

I'm taking people up on their offers.

I have fought and made it through.

I'm still kickin'.

I have a healthy state of mind...I'm no longer in denial.

These last few years with cancer have been the best years of my life.

A sense of relief rushed over me, and I knew I was safe in God's hands.

I am so blessed.

So the three core categories of this model of breast cancer survivor quality of life related to each other. MY ROAD provided the context for MY WALK, and MY WALK described personal strategies for survivorship with a sense of direction that resulted in MY DESTINATION.

Perhaps this model of survivorship developed not only from my interview data, but out of my own consciousness. The HOLDING ON and LETTING GO aspects represented two parts of me that pulled in opposite directions: the need to "get over it" opposed to the need to preserve the one who loved me. Was holding on to my experience with breast cancer a blessing or a curse?

The holding on part felt like George Orwell who had shot and wounded an elephant in India:

"I felt that I had got to put an end to that dreadful noise. It seemed dreadful to see the great beast lying there, powerless to move and yet powerless to die, and not even be able to finish him. I sent back for my small rifle and poured shot after shot into his heart and down his throat. They seemed to make no impression. The tortured gasps continued as steadily as the ticking of a clock."

Towards the end of my research, I had just finished a presentation to a group of cancer survivors at Memorial Hermann Hospital in Houston. I was packing my briefcase, and thinking about lunch. A beautiful woman in her fifties approached me from the back of the room. Her demeanor was polite and demure. She was tall and thin with light brown hair.

She wore her hair long like Laurene had when we first started dating. I noticed her large blue almond-shaped eyes.

"Did your wife attend Waltrip High School?"

"Yes, did you know her?"

"Laurene was my best friend in high school. We were on the drill team together. People said we looked like twins."

"You do look like Laurene...she used to talk about you...the way you did everything together."

"I've had breast cancer for five years. Your model makes sense."

"Thank you."

"Do Neil and Stella still live on Roswell Road?"

"No, they passed away before Laurene."

"They were good people. They let me come along with Laurene to Brownwood once in a while. Stella gave us hard boiled eggs to eat in the back seat of Neil's red truck. Neil was such a kind man."

She disappeared, and I never saw her again.

LESSON THIRTY-ONE

Life is a mysterious process of holding on and letting go.

32.

I hope the women who helped Amphion move the stones
That built the walls of Thebes will help me,
So I won't mistake the facts but only match them exactly.

Dante's Inferno, Canto XXXII

Denise and I decided to get married on Valentine's Day, 2004. Since both of our parents lived near Sarasota, Florida, we chose Sarasota as our wedding location. We figured it would be easier to bring in the children from out of town, than to require our elderly parents to travel. We chose the Sarasota Methodist Church for the ceremony, and the Ritz Carlton for the reception. Our first step involved meeting with a ninety-year-old, semi-retired Methodist minister to plan the wedding.

When Denise married the first time, she was nineteen. She didn't have the wedding she wanted. This time she planned every detail, and recorded her notes in a three-ringed binder. When Dr. Hartsfield glanced at the huge binder, he said, "I only do one wedding." That was it. One wedding. Disappointed, Denise closed her binder. We thought the meeting would be short, since Dr. Hartsfield did only one wedding. We were in for a surprise.

"I've been marrying people for 69 years, and I've learned a few things," he began his monologue:

"First, the two of you are the most important people in your marriage. So there's God and you, and then there's everyone else. But no one else is more important than the two of you—not your friends, not your parents, not your children.

"Second, I've seen more marriages break up from financial problems than any other reason. You need a budget, and you need to decide who writes the checks.

"Third, sex. Now we're Methodists, so you can do about anything you want as long as you do it with love. I mean, if you want to have sex swinging from a chandelier, and you can do it with love in your heart, it's okay as long as you both agree.

"Finally, there is a little boy in every man, and a little girl in every woman. You need to find and honor that child in each other."

Then he took us into the sanctuary for a prayer, and dismissed us. The whole meeting took over 45 minutes, but most of the time was spent counseling us rather than planning the ceremony.

A Husband's Passage Through Cancerland

On February 14, 2004, Denise and I were married in the presence of friends and family. The skies opened up with an afternoon rain storm, so the photographer staged a picture of us kissing under a large umbrella on the veranda of the Ritz. After dinner, the band played the first song for Denise and me. Denise had selected Van Morrison's "Brown Eyed Girl."

Our wedding marked a new life for us. The next day we flew to Hawaii for a two-week honeymoon at the Lodge of Koele Resort on Lanai. We took hikes, played golf, learned trap shooting, and enjoyed reading books in large lounge chairs while sipping cool drinks.

When Denise returned to her work at Pfizer in Kalamazoo, I continued my course work and traveled back and forth to Houston for research, and to San Francisco for classes. I had two more years to go before completing my doctorate. Our life as married couple filled with our blended family, the cat and dog, and new friends. After fifteen years of doing everything herself, Denise began to relax. I began to relax. We had fun together. Denise still mourned the loss of her sister, and I still mourned the loss of Laurene, but we had expanded emotional room to grow as husband and wife.

Following the good preacher's advice, we put each other first. I appreciated the presence of the routines of daily life, without the trips to the cancer clinic and the emergency room, simply having supper together, talking about our daily activities, snuggling in bed before falling asleep, and waking up in the morning to the smell of perking coffee.

The 2004 Atlantic hurricane season struck Florida due to a rare El Niño. More than half of the 16 tropical cyclones brushed or hit the United States, collectively resulting in 3,264 deaths and causing $36.1 billion in damage. Hurricane Charley made landfall in Florida that second week in August. Later in August, Hurricane Frances hit the Bahamas and Florida, leaving severe impact. Hurricane Ivan entered the Gulf of Mexico in early September. The sixth hurricane of the season, Ivan was the size of Texas. Dialysis Centers shut down all along the Florida Coast. Dad's center stayed open, but the facility was overwhelmed. Rather than insisting on keeping his normal schedule, Dad volunteered to receive dialysis at four in the morning.

By early October, Dad had put up and taken down the heavy hurricane shutters three times. He was still not back to his routine schedule of appointments. On October 7, he collapsed at home, and hours later, died in Bon Secours Venice Hospital of cardiac arrest. He was 82. He died holding my mother's hand. Hurricane death statistics did not include Dad. Even though he died sixty years later of a chronic condition created by a war injury, he would never be regarded

A Husband's Passage Through Cancerland

as a casualty of one of the most defining air, land, and sea battles of World War II. Only God knows the total human cost of natural disasters and warfare.

Losing my dad brought me back to the intense grief I had felt a year earlier. From his letters to my Mom during World War II to my most recent phone conversations with him, Dad had showed me how to live each day with joy and gratitude. As a boy, each day my brothers and I would wake up hearing him whistle familiar tunes or sing old Methodist hymns like "Bringing in the Sheaves."

Dad had survived floating mines, enemy PT boats, and a *k* attack, to die a natural death related to a natural disaster. On January 6, 1943, he had written to Mom:

"Once in a while, I'm lucky to have a wonderful dream of you and I together. Someday, darling, we'll be together again and when I wake up, you'll be in my arms, and when I get you in my arms again, lookout!"

For the sixty-two years of their marriage, Dad frequently referred to marriage as entering "the halls of highest human happiness."

So a year that began with new hope, ended with another loss.

LESSON THIRTY-TWO

Life is a series of hops over a landscape of joy and sorrow.

33.

...I said nothing
That entire day and that night,
Until the next day's sun lit up the world.

Dante's Inferno, Canto XXXIII

I showed up for my first retreat at the Vajrapani Institute, a Buddhist retreat center hidden in the mountains near Santa Cruz, California. I parked my rental car, and dragged a roller bag down one side of a ravine, across a stream, and up the other side. I learned later that the Buddhists had closed the footbridge to protect a wasp nest. The roller bag contained what I would normally have taken on a campout: bug spray, binoculars, a compass, a pocketknife, sunglasses, band aids, extra shoelaces, sunscreen, bottled water, two Snickers bars, cigars and a lighter, extra socks, and a floppy hat. I never used a single one of these items. Killing sentient beings with bug spray would have been especially inappropriate, and smoking a cigar was out of the question.

It was November in California, but the temperatures at night in the mountains reached down to the forties. I had signed up for a Saybrook course titled SOCIALLY-ENGAGED SPIRITUALITY. I would spend two weeks in the woods on top of a dark, rainy mountain. I had read the information about the center. Most of our days would be spent in silence, including meals. We would sleep in huts on the mountain above the retreat center and shower outdoors. I tried to imagine what the food would be like, probably no Sloppy Joe's and potato chips. Would they have ice cream?

Redwoods surrounded the low buildings nestled in the mountainside. My 12X16 foot retreat cabin sat at the upper end of a steep path. There were birds in the trees that I had never seen before. Inside the hut, I found a single bed, a meditation cushion, a simple altar, a reading chair, and a small gas stove for making tea. The thermostat read 44 degrees. Outside the hut sat a sink on a weathered redwood deck. From the deck, I could see other huts scattered under the trees. The first night, we were asked to make a pledge not to drink, dance, or have sex while we were there. Buddhist rules to stave off what they called attachment. Toilets sat in a shack about 100 yards further up the mountain where we were told occasional mountain lions lurked.

On the first morning, we began what would be a daily routine for the week. Beginning at seven o'clock in the morning, we meditated for 45 minutes. Walking meditation followed the sitting meditation followed by breakfast in silence. After breakfast, we took a silent break for an hour before beginning silent group meditation. Lunch was served at noon followed by reading discussions and dharma talks. During the talks we were encouraged to sit upright with our legs folded, and to let go of unhelpful thoughts, reactivity, confusion, and disconnections from our body and our heart. Anyone who felt the need to say anything spoke in a soft voice. I wanted to scream. After the dharma talks, we meditated again. Speaking at dinner was optional. Conversations included how do you stay centered when a mosquito goes up your nose? and if I bite this carrot, does the carrot feel pain?

When I found time alone, I began talking to myself. I had thought this course would be a good way to earn easy course credits. I should have known. In college, I had signed up for a first aid course using the same rationale. The woman professor taught the course as if we were medical school students. I had barely escaped with a B. Once again, I had signed up for a greater challenge than I had bargained for. In addition to a massive pile of books and a thick sheaves of readings, we were supposed to learn how to connect our spirituality to social action, to be present to ourselves and others with our full beings, and to be inwardly and outwardly attentive as we descended into nothingness. How could I possibly reach enlightenment without drinking, sex, rock n' roll, and fried food? I couldn't even understand the vocabulary. What was the EIGHTFOLD PATH and the FOUR NOBLE TRUTHS? For me, attachments were documents that you pinned to emails.

Out of the Inferno

I hated the healthy food—hummus, tofu, granola, oatmeal, and endless supplies of veggies. Did I want steamed brown rice, quinoa (does not rhyme with Noah), or millet (does not rhyme with *Olay!*)? Beans or lentils? On the second day, as I nudged my tray through the cafeteria line, a wasp took a sharp bite out of my arm. I yelled reflexively, ***"GODDAMMIT!"***

People looked at me for an instant, and then went on about their business or non-business. A monk dressed in prison orange glanced at me with a disgustingly peaceful look on his face. It made me think how boring perfect happiness must be. Nothing much happens. On the third morning, I traversed the ravine of the wasps and drove my rental car to the nearest town searching for real food. Meditation was hard work, and I needed sustenance.

In Boulder Creek, I found a diner that served poached eggs and corned beef hash, a spiritual setback but oh, so good. I looked longingly at the lunch menu—cheeseburgers and onion rings, an open-faced turkey sandwich with gravy, apple pie a la mode. What would happen to me after two weeks of this? I decided to let go and try, an easy decision on a full stomach.

I looked at the course syllabus while eating the last of my buttered toast slathered with strawberry preserves. To ace this course, all I had to do was to get rid of the Three Poisons: greed, ill will, and delusion.

Then maybe I could help others to be more like me, to be the change I wanted in the world (I began to pick up the lingo). Piece of cake. I ordered four blueberry muffins to take back to my hut, my version of health food.

Each day, walking meditation helped more than sitting. I had always had difficulty sitting still. My long walks in Colorado Springs after Laurene died had been healing, but after four days, the slow pace produced a different effect. As I walked through the rugged terrain, I began to see more of the world around me, but thankfully, no mountain lions.

I spent an hour looking at a small waterfall running through a creek. Embarrassing to admit, I hugged a redwood tree and ran my hand over its gnarly bark. Well, everyone was doing it, so I thought why not? More than anything, no one seemed to care what I did, and I didn't need to impress anyone in any way. I had spent my entire life seeking the approval of others. No one cared.

Halfway through the retreat, Laurene visited me for a second time in a dream. Unlike her first appearance, I was not the center of her attention. She glanced at me sideways as she entered Elevator B at MD Anderson. She winked, then entered the elevator. She looked like she was in a hurry. That was the end of my dream. A few weeks later, I learned that Ellen's breast cancer had metastasized. Ellen had been in the clinic hospital the night that Laurene had appeared to me. Laurene had visited Ellen, not me. The casualness of her appearance assured me. I felt like she was around, but I was no longer the center of her attention. She had other things to do. I didn't feel abandoned by her. We both had work to do. I guess people still have to work in heaven. She had moved on.

By the end of two weeks, I began to regard my body in a new way. I adjusted my clothes for comfort. I wrapped my jacket around my waist when I became too warm. On hot days, I took my shirt off to bask in the sun. I walked barefoot on the mountain paths to feel the dirt under my toes. I no longer worried about the mountain lions. I stopped shaving and left my hair uncombed. My posture improved, and I learned to sit erect with my shoulders back.

At night, I slept more deeply than I had ever slept in my life. I woke refreshed in the morning, eager to spend another day doing nothing. My body felt lighter and my mind emptied. I wanted to follow the syllabus learning objective: "let your ego-self burn out," but I was actually falling in love with *me, me, me, me, me, me*. I wanted to look at my new wild visage in a mirror, but there were no mirrors other than a few puddles when it rained. Were my attempts to follow the Eightfold Path leading me to narcissism? I really didn't care.

I found no telephones, no Internet, and no television. With some helpful tips from the other students, I tried fasting for two days (the cafeteria food facilitated my experiment, because the food offerings were as close to not eating as you could get). For the first time in my life, I ran my hands over my body. I could feel my ribs. I placed my hands on my stomach to feel me breathing. I felt lighter in every way.

The hours of meditation turned out to be a prelude to prayer. I prayed in a new way. I opened myself in a new way. The opening process allowed me to explore how to be useful to others. I was ready to move on, but with a different way of engaging the world. I felt proud of myself, probably not the correct way to feel on your way to Enlightenment.

Driving out of the Santa Cruz Mountains after the retreat, I got lost. I called Denise in Michigan, and told her that I couldn't find my way back to the highway.

"One winding road after another," I said. "I think I'm going to get car sick from the damn curves."

"What do you expect me to do about it?" she said.

"Talk to me so I won't feel lost."

Out of the Inferno

"Didn't they give you a map?"

"The Eightfold Path."

"Sounds confusing."

"Tell me about it."

"So if you're in the mountains, why don't you drive downhill?"

"Great idea."

"Duh."

I am so glad I had married a pilot with common sense. I remembered what her father had told me, "Denise is the one in our family who has her feet on the ground." But he had also taught her how to fly.

On the way to the Oakland Airport, I drove by a shop in Sebastopol advertising natural body care products with the tag line, "Pleasure Heals." *What would Buddha say?*

The next morning, I descended an outdoor staircase from my second floor motel room near the Oakland airport. A homeless man, carrying a large green plastic bag, popped out from behind the staircase. He made a move towards me with his hand out, and said he was hungry. I asked him if he wanted to have breakfast with me, but he ran away. Maybe I looked too wild. He would have enjoyed what I ordered for breakfast.

LESSON THIRTY-THREE

Spiritual practice leads to service.

34.

My teacher and I entered that secluded passage
That would lead us back to the lit world.
Not wanting to waste time resting, we climbed—
Him first, then me—until we came to a round opening
Through which I saw some of the beautiful things
That come with Heaven. And we walked out
To once again catch sight of the stars.

Dante's Inferno, Canto XXXIV

I am standing in front of Laurene's niche in the memorial garden on a feeder road bordering Texas Highway 45, the highway we had traveled from home to the clinic and back for a decade, the highway with the billboard still shouting GALLERY FURNITURE SAVES YOU MONEY! Standing there brought to mind the little spaces of our world during those years—our favorite restaurants, our pew at the back of the sanctuary, the lilies in our garden near the magnolia tree, the springtime fields of bluebonnets and Indian Paintbrush near Brennan, the trampoline in our backyard once bounced upon by now grown little girls.

Wind gusts rustle through the tops of the cypress trees like waves, and the dark brown leaves on the ground whirl in circles. Rain begins to fall from a tar black sky. Water drops follow each other down tear trails on the granite memorial wall. I unclench my hands, and move my fingers lightly over the face of Laurene's plaque. I brush away the raindrops to read the inscription we had placed under her name: OUR BLUEBONNET ANGEL. I hear traffic zoom by on the slick pavement. I walk back to the parking lot. Headlights glitter from the road. I hop in my truck, and the wind slams the door on my seat belt. I reopen the door, and the wind slams the door again.

One of my research participants summed up where I had arrived:

"I am now, after a long struggle, surprisingly happy in the crooked, sturdy little shelter I've built for myself in the wastes of CANCERLAND."

While CANCERLAND describes my journey through a cancer inferno, like Dante Alighieri, my point of arrival after the journey had taken a different character. Dante had developed new understandings of compassion and justice, good and evil, pride and humility, anger and fear. So had I.

During my passage through CANCERLAND I had learned how to live my life in a different way: to live with confusion and puzzlement, to give and receive help and love, to feel both competent and useless, to make bad decisions as well as good ones, to be in awe of the mastery of others and aware of my imperfections, to get tangled up in questions of right and wrong, to bear suffering alone and without understanding, to experience the mysteries of anger and joy, the mixtures of hope, despair, fear, loneliness, the unrelenting burden of grief, the inevitability of death, and a new understanding of God.

I had grown into a new stage of adulthood. By traveling through CANCERLAND, I had entered what Belle, a character in *Abide with Me* by Elizabeth Strout, calls GROWN UP LAND. At the end of the novel, Belle says to Tyler, "Meanwhile, welcome to grown-up land."

During this time, the grandchildren that Laurene had hoped to see have been born—four boys and four girls. Denise and I have also lost her father and mother, and my father and mother have died. We continue to live through an unending process of holding on and letting go, of birth and death, like living through the seasons—fall, winter, spring, summer, and fall again—experiencing the changes in weather and the whole of nature. Like the legendary phoenix of the ancient Egyptians, a bird consumed by its own fire, we keep struggling each day to rise refreshed from our own ashes. OUT OF THE INFERNO. That's what people do. That's what we all do. The best we can.

My journey with breast cancer remains rooted deep in my consciousness. I will never lose the emotional attachment to the journey or the drastic changes it caused in my life. But when the journey reappears in one way or the other, I don't regard the appearance as an unwanted resurrection or something I need to rebury. It would be like throwing water on a fire that never goes out. I'm simply aware, like the giving or receiving of unconditional love. I have forgiven myself for the things I did awkwardly and wrong, and I appreciate what I did skillfully and well. And when I see suffering around me, it seems like a well-worn road to travel with compassion, kindness, and love.

Every day I pray for a cure for breast cancer, or a way to manage cancer as a chronic but treatable condition. I know that my wife and daughters, my sister-in-laws or daughters-in-law, or my granddaughters could be diagnosed with breast cancer, or even the men in my life. I don't want to forget about breast cancer anymore than I want to forget about Laurene, but now I can face the future without bitterness or self-pity. I have let go of the anxiety in favor of new love and the work I want to do. The swings of my personal pendulum have modulated.

I attended my last meeting with the Sisters Network. Three years had passed since I first attended their Saturday support group meeting, three years since Gladys had called to invite me back. My dissertation was about to be published. Over 250 women had developed quality of life action plans based on my survivorship model. The Houston Breast Cancer Group Leaders Network had started to meet without me. At the end of the Sisters meeting, the pastor prayed for me. Her prayer ended this way: "As Randy finishes his doctoral work, may he continue to live in ways that lead to the highest degree anyone can receive as a son of God."

Laurene's memory is no longer contained in picture boxes. I see her in the eyes of the ones I love, and through the work I do. I see her in day-to-day experience, and I see her in myself. I don't remember her so much as I relive her. Even though my heart remains peopled with absences, the ones who have passed on, my heart is undivided and free to love.

Deep love can transfer to others. It is God-like and boundless, ready for sacrifice. I love and appreciate Denise as if she were my one and only love from the beginning, and if anything, I love her with more gratitude for regaining what I had lost. There is no such thing as one true love, or one love that is more real than another.

Four years ago, I started to write. Floodgates of words flowed onto the pages. Unblocked from my life script of making a living, and free of my drives to be secure, safe, and predictable, I began to trust myself and trust the value of what I had to say to others. I began by filling in the blank pages of the journal that Laurene had given to me when she was first diagnosed. Over the last four years, I have written two novels, a collection of poetry, essays, short stories, a play, a fable, and this memoir. Writing has introduced me to a new way of seeing the world and being myself.

Both novels involve the everyday life of protagonist widowers who make mistakes and get into trouble of their own doing.

Crooked River tells the story of laid-off Rebecca Randall who finds love, adventure, and a sense of belonging in northern Michigan when she decides to visit her father, a war-damaged recluse, who lives in a cabin on Devil's Elbow, a sharp bend in the Crooked River. Finding a home serves as a major theme.

The Lawnmower Club, a playful foray into magical realism, creates a curmudgeonly character named Leo Zitzelberger who loses his wife, his house, and his yard, and proceeds to create his version of paradise on earth by purchasing a bankrupt golf course, and selling memberships to men like himself who are obsessed with cutting grass. A rogue cougar, a social worker, and a local resorter try to thwart his efforts. Finding a home provides the plot.

Neither narrative leads to miraculous redemptions, but rather each character finds a happy landing place in the watery landscape of northern Michigan.

Writing the novels helped release my grief, but writing the memoir has helped me in ways that nothing else could do. Rather than burying my feelings in fiction, telling Laurene's true story, and the true stories of others, has freed me from the oppression of those long years. I no longer try to put that part of my life away for keeps or get over it. Life after Laurene has become a way of surrendering without defeat, a way of entering new relationships without having to give up the old, a way of living in the sunshine rather than the twilight.

This memoir has been a gift. The writing has released joy, vitality, meaning, and purpose in me. I don't know many people who think they have succeeded as caregivers, and I don't feel that way either. I don't feel like an expert.

There is so much you can do, but so much that you cannot do. You cannot be your spouse's doctor, therapist, spiritual advisor, and support group. You cannot make the illness go away, or protect against the side effects. People call you a saint when you know you're not, and most of the time you're simply ignored. I have no special wisdom. The lessons have come out of my experience. The lessons may or may not help others. They are my perspective.

These days I stand and look at Laurene in the faces of my children and grandchildren, and occasionally I run across artifacts of her life—a favorite bookmark, a tiny hinged frame of Jennifer and Meredith's school pictures, candlesticks from our trip to the Murano Glass Factory, Neil's Father of the Year plaque, a photograph of Laurene's uncle riding a bull in a rodeo, and the neatly labeled keepsake boxes.

I'm always grateful to recover something of what I lost in the exchange of life. The weight of the physical artifacts comforts me, and validates those difficult years.

When we married, Denise carried her own artifacts with her—her father's flight book, his Navy dress uniform, her grandmother's Maxfield Parrish illustrations, her costume sketches from college drama class, a framed *Ladies' Home Journal* advertisement for West Electric Hair Curlers, invented by her great grandfather, pictures of her Aunt Dorothy and Uncle Dave, shelves of Fiesta and Hall pottery, Dana's doll house, and a roomful of Dana's stuffed animals.

We all carry our past forward, and face the future as best we can. We keep forming new lives out of the raw materials of our past. We walk into a new story, carrying the old stories in a bag strapped like a sack of memories across our shoulders.

Tonight I'm finished and going to bed. I will turn to what Josie, my granddaughter, calls the good dream side of the pillow. But first I have to tell Denise a bedtime story. The little girl in her wants a new story every night. I know that I only need to get the story started, because she prefers to do the endings.

It had taken Dante and Virgil 24 hours from Good Friday evening to Holy Saturday evening to traverse the nine circles of Hell. When they exited at the foot of Mount Purgatory, Easter Monday dawned. As they looked at the early morning sky to once again catch sight of the stars, the journey had only begun.

LESSON THIRTY-FOUR

There is no such thing as starting over.

ACKNOWLEDGEMENTS

Thanks to readers who have supported my new career as a writer over the last ten years, especially Karen Langs at McLean & Eakin Book Store in Petoskey, Michigan, and my writing group buddies: Al Sevener, Rose Dobrez, Gary Edwards, Kenn Grimes, Jessica Holmann, Tom Johnson, Mary Koppel, Sheri and Wendy Lawler, Ellen Reddy, Sara Sabourin, Al Sevener, Laura Sprague, Peggy Vork-Zambory, Chris Weston, and Matt Ziselman.

Thanks to Linda Yarger, librarian at MD ANDERSON and breast cancer survivor. Linda supported Laurene and me over the ten years of Laurene's treatment, helped me with my doctoral studies of breast cancer support groups, and reviewed this book for accuracy and precision, particularly on medical subjects that were over my head.

Thanks to my editor, Wade Rouse, best-selling memoirist and author of THE CHARM BRACELET (St. Martin's Press), written under the pen name Viola Shipman as a tribute to his grandmother. Wade never stopped insisting that I share my story with a wider audience.

Thanks to Mike Schlitt, founder of the CHARLEVOIX PHOTOGRAPHY CLUB, for his photographic art, and to Angela Hoy and Todd Engel for their publishing and cover design expertise at BOOKLOCKER.COM, INC.

And love, appreciation, and admiration to Denise Evans, my wife, cheerleader, literary critic, source of sunshine, and the one without whom I would be lost.

CPSIA information can be obtained
at www.ICGtesting.com
Printed in the USA
FSOW02n1143100616
21392FS